# BDJ Clinician's Guides

This series enables clinicians at all stages of their careers to remain well informed and up to date on key topics across all fields of clinical dentistry. Each volume is superbly illustrated and provides concise, highly practical guidance and solutions. The authors are recognised experts in the subjects that they address. The *BDJ Clinician's Guides* are trusted companions, designed to meet the needs of a wide readership. Like the *British Dental Journal* itself, they offer support for undergraduates and newly qualified, while serving as refreshers for more experienced clinicians. In addition they are valued as excellent learning aids for postgraduate students.

The BDJ Clinicians' Guides are produced in collaboration with the British Dental Association, the UK's trade union and professional association for dentists.

Craig Barclay
Editor

# Oral Implantology: Assessment to Maintenance

Springer

*Editor*
Craig Barclay
Restorative Dentistry
University Dental Hospital of Manchester
Manchester, UK

ISSN 2523-3327 ISSN 2523-3335 (electronic)
BDJ Clinician's Guides
ISBN 978-3-031-55240-3 ISBN 978-3-031-55241-0 (eBook)
https://doi.org/10.1007/978-3-031-55241-0



This Springer imprint is published by the registered company Springer Nature Switzerland AG
The registered company address is: Gewerbestrasse 11, 6330 Cham, Switzerland

# Foreword

This is a timely book designed for general dentists with an interest in implants. In fact, this book ought to be compulsory reading for anyone who wants to work with oral implants. In the past, we had very thorough week-long training courses for implantologists to-be, whereas today many start working in this field without much knowledge, in many cases resulting in unnecessarily poor clinical outcomes. The importance of the human factor for implant problems is substantial and has been known for many years; Ross Bryant demonstrated in his Ph.D. thesis in 2001 that surgeons and restorative dentists active at the University of Toronto had substantial differences in average marginal bone loss, despite using the same implant type in similar patient population. A patient treated by the least optimal surgeon, followed by actions by the poorest restorative dentist displayed an average marginal bone loss (MBL) of 2 mm in contrast to those handled by the best pair of colleagues where the total MBL was of the order of 0.2 mm.

Most chapters in this book have a rather fragmentary list of references which is quite understandable in a book aimed for clinicians; overloading the message with a lot of references does not make reading easier. There are always matters that can be discussed, and let me start with one of the most common terms in implant dentistry, even used in the title of Chap. 1, 'dental implants'. Writing it like this somehow gives the impression that we are referring to teeth. Oral implants would be a much more suitable term. Chapters 2, 3, and 4 discuss the most important matters, including the relatively common presence of an anterior loop of the mandibular nerve and the importance of carefully listening to patients and actively asking them about any medicines they may be taking. The anterior loop of the mandibular nerve may give rise to patient pain that is impossible to treat clinically. We have sectioned such implants after needed removal and found nerves in every thread of the implant which is a clear pathological finding and most likely explained by mandibular nerve loops. A proper anamnesis is most important since the patient history is something to learn from for the dentist in general. We need information of all pharmaceutical products taken by the patient. I am referring to anti-depressants such as serotonin inhibitors that may prevent osseointegration if the patients take them at the time of surgery or $H_2$ antagonists that may cause marginal bone loss and even implant failure if consumed at any time.

I was not aware that subperiosteal implants (they are, in fact, no implants since retention is achieved by securing soft tissue layers above metal constructions) have had a renaissance in severely resorbed clinical cases. The so-called subs were not the worst of older constructions used, and there were even some long-term clinical reports published in the past. Personally, I may still prefer short implants or grafting procedures to solve such cases, but I am a most conservative osseointegrationist and provided that subs are backed by improved clinical results compared to the other alternatives for severely resorbed patients they are here to stay.

The so-called intramobile elements proved ineffective with the IMZ implant, as discussed in Chap. 8. However, since a photograph of such implants is presented, we must remember that they were catastrophic designs that lost bone in an unacceptable manner and should never have been used clinically with or without the intramobile elements. It is excellent that Chap. 9 provides a critical discussion of the use of probes. Those who tried to probe Brånemark's implant in the good old days would have had to look for a new job the next day. As pointed out by Coli (who is rightfully quoted), probing teeth may be acceptable, but not so with implants.

Having said this, there is admittedly one category of dentists who would not regard even the possibility of not using probes, regardless of whether the patient has only natural teeth or only implants. One can nevertheless be somewhat critical of this, as there have been no studies attempting to analyse whether probed implants fared as well as non-probed ones in the long run.

In Chap. 10, various clinical results are quoted, which is fine. Today, we see no difference between maxillary and mandibular long-term outcome, and we have approximately 15 different full 10-year studies of moderately rough surfaces published, indicative of a limited failure rate of between 1% and 4%. Admittedly, if poorly trained clinicians were to use poorly documented implant systems, failures and other problems would likely be much more substantial than the figures quoted above.

An assumed implant plague in the form of the so-called peri-implantitis has allegedly been threatening an enormous number of implants. In the light of the very good long-term results reported with oral implants with the great majority of the failures seen occurring in the first few years, the least one can say is that problems with this disease have been grossly exaggerated in the literature. In reality, as pointed out in Chap. 9, marginal bone loss is not solely dependent on bacteria. Chap. 11 presents one illustration with numerous listed subfactors which may cause marginal bone loss, the great majority of those being quite unrelated to bacteria. The mechanism of marginal bone loss lies instead with the immune system that controls the combined action of osteoblasts and osteoclasts. This is an example of aseptic bone loss, which we generally see when the immune system maintains control over bacterial attacks. However, when too much combined trauma occurs, it may force the immune system to surrender which opens up for secondary bacterial attacks on failing implants. The importance of the immune system in osseointegration as well as in perturbation of osseointegration could have been stressed a bit in this book, but admittedly this is in the present research frontier and as of yet not in the mind of every clinician.

If you are a non-specialized clinician or an implant novice and have not purchased this book yet, do so now. It will be necessary reading to learn more about the fascinating use of oral implants, and both you and your patients will benefit from the accumulated knowledge herein.

Department of Biomaterials
University of Gothenburg
Gothenburg, Sweden

Tomas Albrektsson

# Contents

# 1 What is an Oral Implant?

Craig Barclay

An endosteal dental implant is an artificial tooth root, normally made of titanium, which is inserted into the alveolar bone and used prosthodontically to facilitate the replacement of missing teeth. Historically, various materials have been inserted into the jawbone as artificial roots, dating back to around 2000 BC in ancient China, where carved bamboo pegs were used as early versions of dental implants to replace the missing teeth. The first recorded use of metal within the jaw bones was noted in the maxilla of an Egyptian king around 1000 BC. However, it was not clear if the copper peg found hammered into the maxilla was placed during his lifetime as a tooth replacement or placed after his death.

In 1952, while examining the femur bone of a rabbit, a Swedish physician and morphologist named P-I Branemark discovered that the titanium case of the microscope lens adhered to the bone. He hypothesized that this fusion, later named osseointegration, could be useful in the fields of both dentistry and orthopaedics. The first titanium oral implant was placed in a human in 1965 by P-I Branemark's team, and the first peer-reviewed paper was published in 1977 [1].

Oral implants have evolved with changes to shape, surfaces and connection type [2]. In 1992, Misch and Misch described generic prosthetic component terminology, describing an oral implant as any material or device placed in and/or on oral tissues to support an oral prosthesis. They classified oral implants as being endosseous (within the bone), subperiosteal (beneath the periosteum), transosteal (through the bone), intramucosal (within the mucosa) and endodontic (within the root canal system of a tooth). The majority of endosseous (also known as endosteal) oral implants are made of pure titanium, which is commercially available in four grades, defined by the amount of carbon, nitrogen, oxygen and iron contained [3].

The various terms used in the early 1990s by Misch still apply today and help dentists describe the various components required in this discipline (Fig. 1.1).

---

C. Barclay (✉)
Restorative Dentistry/Oral Rehabilitation, Manchester Foundation Trust, Manchester, UK
e-mail: Craig.Barclay@mft.nhs.uk



C. Barclay (ed.), *Oral Implantology: Assessment to Maintenance*, BDJ Clinician's Guides, https://doi.org/10.1007/978-3-031-55241-0_1

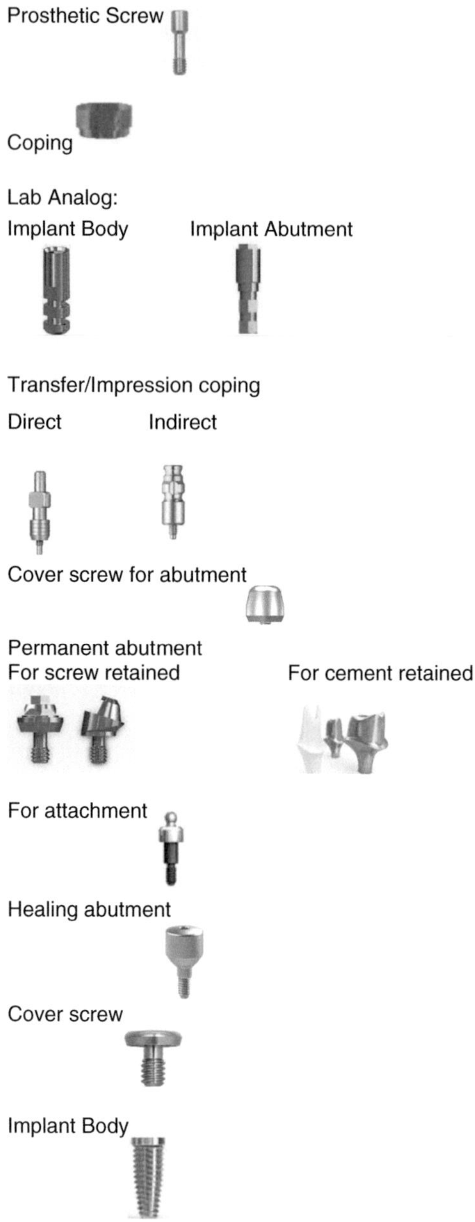


**Fig. 1.1** Dental implant components

Where possible, dentists strive to return patients to full aesthetic and functional dental health. Over the last 50 years, the use of endosteal oral implants has allowed a fixed and removable option to be provided for patients following natural tooth loss. The challenge for us as dentists is to be able to both identify the implant system used and be able to maintain that implant system effectively. It is estimated that there are around 150 dental companies worldwide that manufacture oral implants with over 500 different dental implant systems currently available. In 2021, it was estimated that 18 million oral implants were sold. This can make identification of a placed dental implant clinically challenging and consequently complicate one's ability to be able to access the correct implant components if replacement parts are required. However, with digital scanners and computer-aided-design/computer-aided-manufacturing (CAD/CAM) technologies, it is now possible to generate bespoke implant components if required.

Various body shapes of endosteal implants have been designed over the years, ranging from bullet-shaped, stepped, cylindrical and tapered (Fig. 1.2). Most modern implants are threaded with different pitches and shapes of threads (Fig. 1.3). In

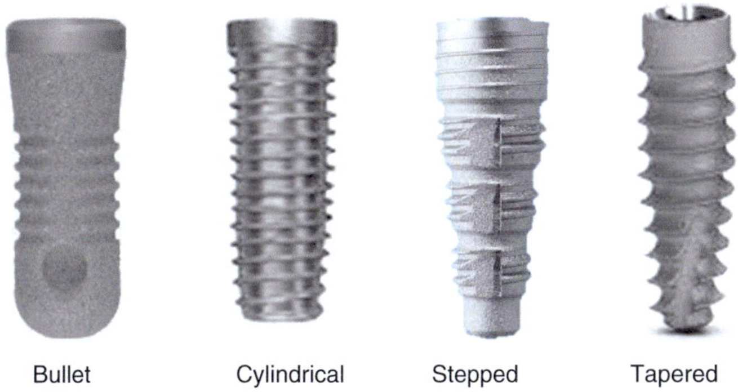


**Fig. 1.2** Shapes of dental implants

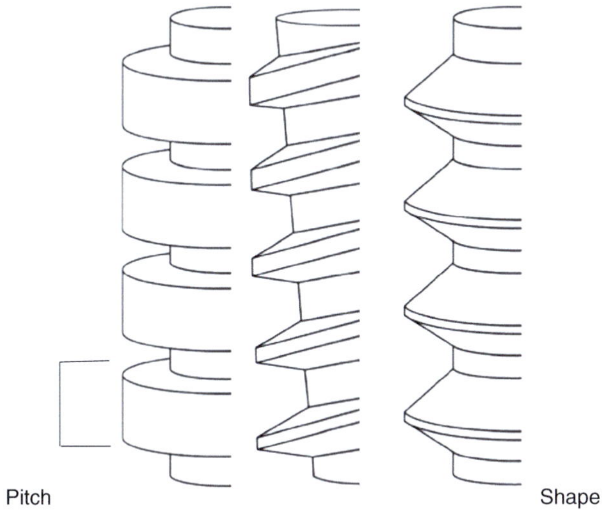


**Fig. 1.3** Pitch and shape of thread

vivo studies indicate that stress distribution varies with the thread shape. Thread pitch is defined as the distance between two neighbouring threads, measured on the same side of the axis.

Another method used to not only increase the surface area of the oral implant but also alter bone apposition is surface topography. Most oral implants are machined from titanium and then the surface is either cleaned after machining, altered by various removal processes or added with additional layers. Machined, or as sometimes referred to as polished, oral implants have a surface roughness (Sa) of around 0.9 μm, as opposed to some new implant surfaces that have been sandblasted and had additions to the surface, resulting in an Sa value of over 1.7 μm.

Oral implant surfaces can therefore be machined, alumina oxide-blasted, plasma-sprayed, electrolytic-etched, coated with hydroxyapetite or even enhanced with various nano-particles in the newest generation. All these surface preparations can, in theory, alter the adherence of the salivary pellicle and plaque to the implant surface as well as have beneficial effects in terms of integration.

The connection type of an oral implant is the method by which the superstructure is connected to the body of the oral implant. An implant can be either in one piece or two pieces where an abutment is fitted to the body of the implant (Fig. 1.4). External and internal connections can have several different design shapes and configurations, as shown in Fig. 1.5.

Most endosteal implants are not a single piece and therefore either rely on an abutment to be connected, onto which the prosthesis is attached, or the prosthesis is connected directly to the implant. When the prosthesis is connected directly to the implant, this is called a fixture-level restoration; if the prosthesis is connected via an abutment, this is called an abutment-level restoration (Fig. 1.6).

**Advantages of Abutment-Supported Prostheses**

- If implants are not parallel to each other, angulated abutments can adjust for this.
- Prefabricated abutments are available for a screw-retained prosthesis, and prefabricated and custom abutments can be fabricated for a cemented prosthesis.
- Placement of abutments permits the abutment–prosthesis interface to be placed sub- or supra-crestal, making management of the soft tissues more controlled.
- Removal and placement of an abutment-supported prosthesis is more comfortable for the patient compared to an implant-supported prosthesis.

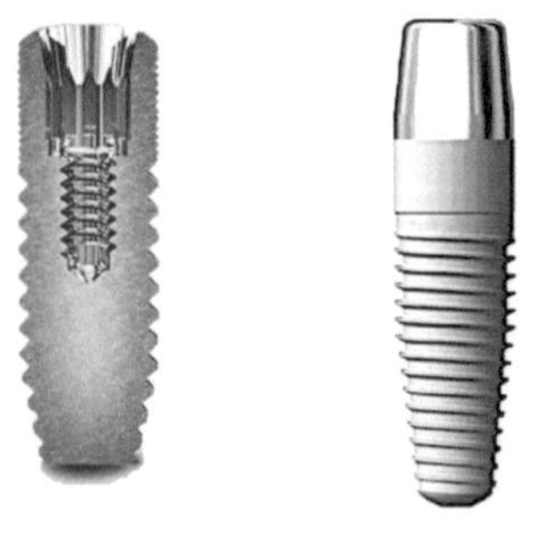


**Fig. 1.4** One- or two-piece dental implants

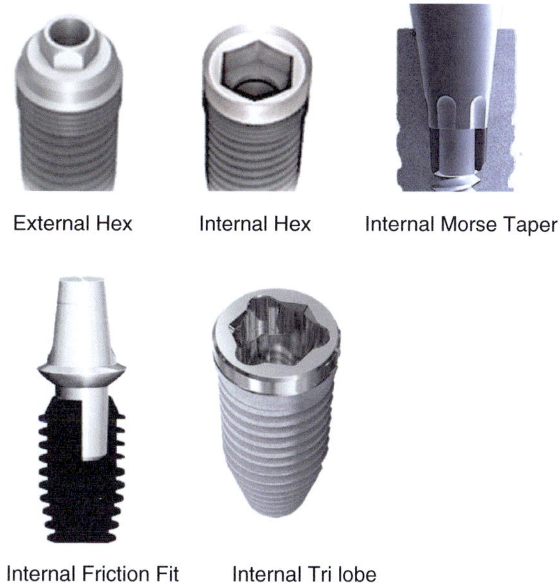


**Fig. 1.5** Variety of connection types

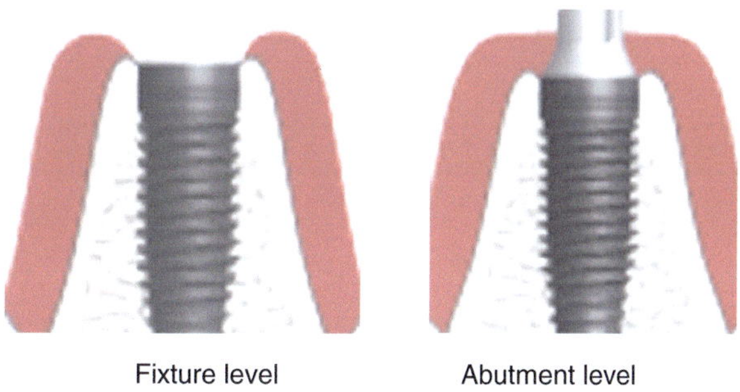


**Fig. 1.6** The superstructure is either connected direct to the implant (fixture-level) or via a connection (abutment-level)

**Advantages of Implant-Supported Prosthesis**

- When there is limited inter-arch space, this type of prosthesis allows for the necessary space for the prosthesis.
- There is only one retentive mechanism to check.

A prosthesis connection to the oral implant can be either fixed or removable (Fig. 1.7). A fixed prosthesis is screw- or cement-retained (Fig. 1.8). The scientific literature suggests that fixed implant restorations require less maintenance compared to removable implant prostheses [4].

A removable implant prosthesis can be attached to the implants by a variety of attachment methods. The most common methods of denture retention utilizing implants are studs, locators, magnets and bars (Fig. 1.9)

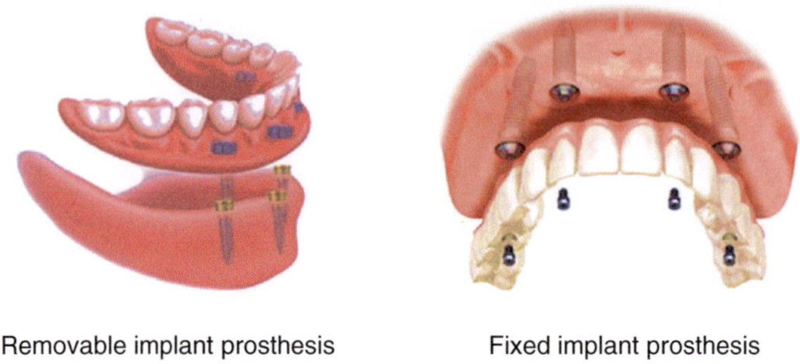


**Fig. 1.7** The superstructure can either be removed or fixed to the dental implants

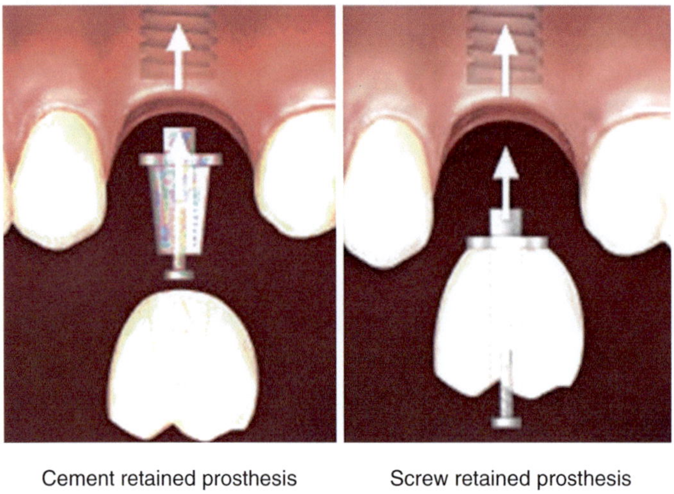


**Fig. 1.8** A fixed prosthesis can be either screw- or cement-retained [5]

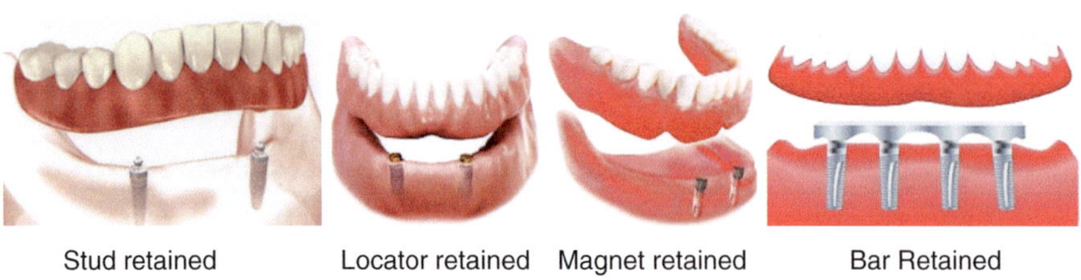


**Fig. 1.9** Removable denture attachments to dental implants

Irrespective of the method of attachment, it is good practice to take a baseline radiograph of bone levels around the implants on the first day of loading, to allow future assessment and comparison of bone levels. It is also important, where possible, to give the patient some form of an implant passport so that in the future the patient is aware of the implant system, the implant size and width and the method of attachment used. This will enable any dentist who then sees this patient to have a starting point in terms of the implant system present intra-orally.

## References

1. Branemark P-I, Hansson B-O, Adell R, Breine U, Lindstrom J, Hallen O, Ohman A. Osseointegrated implants in the treatment of the edentulous jaw. Experience from a 10-year period. Scand J Plast Reconstr Surg Suppl. 1977;16:1–132.
2. Misch CE, Misch CM. Generic terminology for endosseous implant prosthodontics. J Prosthet Dent. 1992;68:809–12.
3. Natali AN, editor. Dental biomechanics. London/New York: Taylor & Francis; 2003. p. 69–87, 273 pp., ISBN 978-0-415-30666-9.
4. Walton JN, MacEntee MI. Problems with prostheses on implants: a retrospective study. J Prosthet Dent. 1994;71:283–8.
5. Wittneben J-G, Joda T, Weber H-P, Brägger U. Screw retained vs. cement retained implant-supported fixed dental prosthesis. Periodontology 2000. 2017;73:141–51.

# Case Selection/Indications for Implant Treatment

# 2

Julian Yates

The clinical examination is undertaken to assess the suitability of the patient for treatment and to devise a patient-centred management plan before, during, and after implant surgery. During the clinical examination, pertinent issues related to potential implant treatment should be identified and used not only to advise the patient, but also to aid the clinician in planning for surgery. Furthermore, it may also highlight existing problems or features that in certain circumstances may be thought to be attributed to implant treatment, when in fact they are not. Important findings may include pre-existing oral infections, dental pathology (including periodontal disease), facial swellings or temporomandibular joint disorders. Furthermore, a functional exam should be undertaken to determine any parafunctional habits that can be used to advise the patient for or against any procedure or planned prosthesis [1, 2].

Intra-oral and extra-oral examination form the basis for every surgical case, and the findings should be used to determine the shape, size, and position of the implants to be used, and the type of prosthesis provided.

## 2.1 Radiographic Assessment

Radiographic assessment in implant dentistry plays an essential role in assessing the available bone, treatment planning, and also reviewing the long-term stability of hard tissues once treatment has been completed. In order to plan for optimal treatment and a successful outcome, the quantity and quality of bone need to be assessed to determine the correct implant position in relation to the position and design of the prosthesis required. Radiographic imaging is also needed to assess the presence of dental disease, the condition of existing natural teeth, and position of important

J. Yates (✉)
Oral Surgery, Division of Dentistry, School of Medical Sciences, University of Manchester, Manchester, UK
e-mail: julian.yates@manchester.ac.uk



C. Barclay (ed.), *Oral Implantology: Assessment to Maintenance*, BDJ Clinician's Guides, https://doi.org/10.1007/978-3-031-55241-0_2

anatomical structures where implant placement is planned, all of which may influence the treatment proposed.

There is no doubt regarding the value of the various imaging methods used in implant dentistry. However, due to the limited evidence available, there is significant debate in relation to the selection criteria for the correct imaging used in individual clinical situations, and at which points along the treatment pathway and for how long after completion follow-up radiographs should be taken.

Whilst a thorough clinical examination, in addition to 2D radiographic imaging, may be adequate for simple cases, sectional or 3D imaging is commonly recommended in complex cases. Furthermore, 3D radiological techniques may be used to construct surgical guides or stents and to improve the accuracy of implant placement or even in the design and manufacture of prostheses, immediate or otherwise.

Baseline radiographic examination is recommended after the prosthodontic phase of treatment to assess marginal bone levels, to check on the fitting of the implant and prosthetic components, and to allow comparison of hard tissues should problems arise at a later date.

## 2.2 Anatomical Considerations

A comprehensive knowledge of oral anatomy is needed to undertake safe and effective implant treatment/surgery, as there are anatomical structures relevant to the dental implantologist that must be considered prior to any treatment. A sound knowledge of the relationships of muscles, blood supply, foramina, and nerves that may be encountered during implant treatment need to be understood, and caution must be exercised when performing surgery in certain regions of the oral cavity. Additional consideration must also be given to changes in hard and soft tissue anatomy following tooth extraction/loss, as this may impact on the provision of dental implants.

### 2.2.1 Anatomical Considerations in the Mandible

*Inferior Alveolar Nerve:* The mandibular branch of the trigeminal nerve gives rise to the inferior alveolar nerve (IAN). It enters the mandibular canal on the medial surface of the ramus of the mandible immediately adjacent to the lingula. The mandibular canal is approximately 3–4 mm in diameter whilst the nerve itself is approximately 2–3 mm thick [3]. As with most peripheral nerves, it is accompanied by an artery, a vein, and often lymphatic vessels. The vessels lie on the surface of the nerve as it traverses through the mandibular canal anteriorly, but their position in relation to the nerve varies within the mandibular canal.

When preparing an osteotomy for implant placement over the mandibular canal, cortical bone is penetrated first, which is then followed by preparation within the softer cancellous bone. Whilst the mandibular canal is usually surrounded by hard cortical bone and affords some protection to the IAN, inadvertent penetration into the canal may cause damage to both the nerve and/or vessels, therefore causing altered sensation to the ipsilateral teeth, lip, and chin. When undertaking implant placement in the posterior mandible, clinicians should not rely on tactile feel alone to determine the position of the mandibular canal, as inconsistencies in the density of the bone when preparing the osteotomy will more than likely lead to difficulties in assessing the true position of the drill in relation to the nerve. Therefore, accurate planning must be undertaken, including precise radiographic (2D or CBCT) assessment in order to prevent such injuries. It should be remembered that in approximately 25% of the patients the walls of the mandibular canal cannot be clearly identified in the premolar and molar regions on standard 2D periapical radiographs. In such cases, it is recommended that an Orthopantomogram (OPT) with adjustments for magnification or Cone-beam computed tomography (CBCT) imaging are undertaken to visualize the position of the nerve in relation to the height available for implant selection and osteotomy preparation. Implant placement in the posterior mandible should not be undertaken in cases where the position of the IAN has not been determined.

Planning for accurate implant placement in the posterior mandible is shown in Fig. 2.1. Furthermore, additional safety devices, including the use of drill marks, drill stops and/or surgical guides for preparing osteotomies for specific implant lengths in this region of the mouth, may also be of some benefit.

*Mental Foramen and Nerve:* The position of the mental foramen differs in both the horizontal and vertical planes, and these variations can be significant. Horizontally, the foramen is most commonly situated immediately adjacent to the apices of the second mandibular premolar tooth; however, it may be situated more anteriorly towards the canine or more posteriorly towards the first molar in some cases. The position of the foramen also varies in the vertical plane. Various studies have reported that in the first and second premolar region the mental foramen was situated superior to the tooth apex in approximately 25–40% of cases, at the apex in 15% of cases, and inferior to the apex in 60–45% of the cases, respectively. Therefore, when preparing an osteotomy for implant placement in the premolar region, extreme care must be taken as the emergence of the mental foramen and

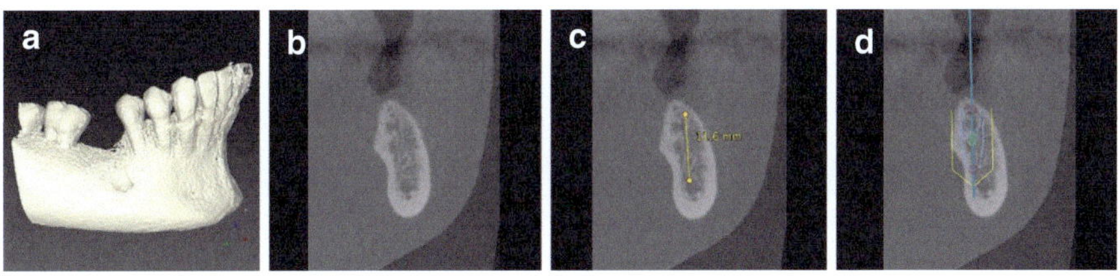


**Fig. 2.1** CBCT images demonstrating planning for implant placement in the posterior mandible in order to avoid iatrogenic damage to the inferior alveolar nerve (IAN)—(**a**) 3D reconstructed image of the right posterior mandible from a CBCT scan; (**b**) cross-sectional image of the mandible immediately distal to the mental foramen; (**c**) measurement of the distance from the alveolar crest to superior border of the IAN; (**d**) planned position and length of the dental implant above the IAN (note the safety margin placed around the planned osteotomy site to further reduce the risk of nerve injury)

nerve may be positioned coronal to the expected apex of the teeth in approximately 25–40% of the cases [4–6].

Additional consideration should also be given when undertaking treatment in areas of bony atrophy and when performing bilateral procedures, as the position of the nerve may well be asymmetrical and not comparable to the contra-lateral side.

*Anterior Loop of the Mental Nerve:* An additional consideration when assessing the position of the IAN when it emerges from the mental foramen is the anterior loop of the mental nerve and the presence of the intra-medullary incisive branch. Frequently the nerve deviates inferiorly and anteriorly in relation to the foramen prior to its emergence from the mandible. Although present, there are conflicting reports in relation to the size and incidence of the anterior loop due to the different criteria used to characterize it, and the difficulty in isolating and identifying the incisive branch of the IAN. Reports have suggested the presence of an anterior loop in approximately 25–35% of cases, depending on radiographic or clinical evidence, and that the diameter of the anterior loop can vary from 1 to 3 mm and extend anteriorly from the mental foramen by up to 6–7 mm [7]. Given the potential for implant insertion into the inter-foramina space, care must be taken not only with raising any mucoperiosteal flap but also when undertaking osteotomy preparation and placing implants in this region. (Fig. 2.2)

In cases where the mandible is edentulous, there can be extreme variation in the position of the mental foramen, and these must be anticipated prior to any surgery. Relative to its position in dentate patients, the position can be different in both the vertical and horizontal plane in edentulous patients due to hard tissue changes that can occur following tooth loss, and in extreme cases it can even be present supra-crestally. (Fig. 2.3)

*Sub-Mental and Sub-Lingual Arteries:* The sub-mental and sub-lingual arteries are continuations of the facial and lingual arteries, respectively (Fig. 2.4).

The sub-lingual artery is found superior to the mylohyoid muscle, whilst the sub-mental artery frequently traverses inferiorly to the mylohyoid muscle. A consistent

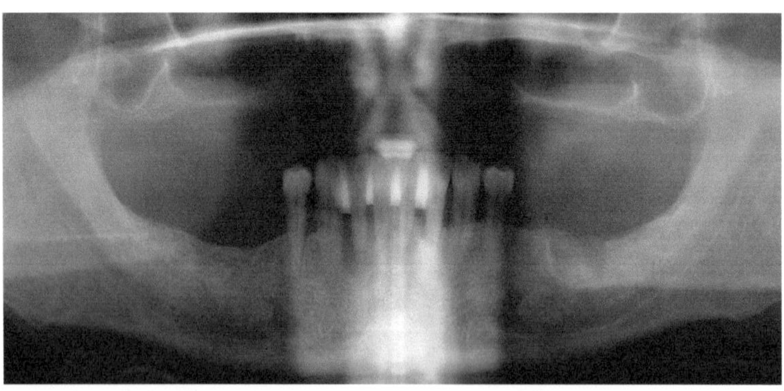

**Fig. 2.2** OPT radiograph highlighting the position of the left and right inferior alveolar nerves with the presence of anterior loops prior to the emergence of the mental nerve. These may encroach on the planned implant placement in the inter-foramina space

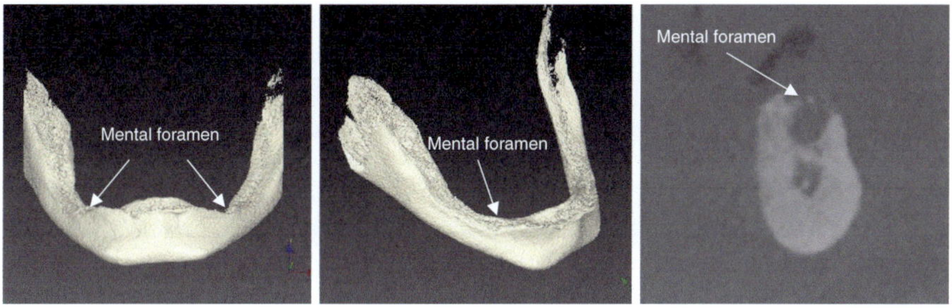


**Fig. 2.3** CBCT images demonstrating the presence of the mental foramen in an atrophic mandible (**a**) anterior view of 3D reconstructed image of the mandible illustrating the position of the mental foramen on the superior aspect of the alveolus; (**b**) oblique view of 3D reconstructed image of the mandible at the site of the right mental foramen; (**c**) cross-sectional image at the site of the right mental foramen—note the exit of the mental nerve on the superior aspect of the alveolar ridge

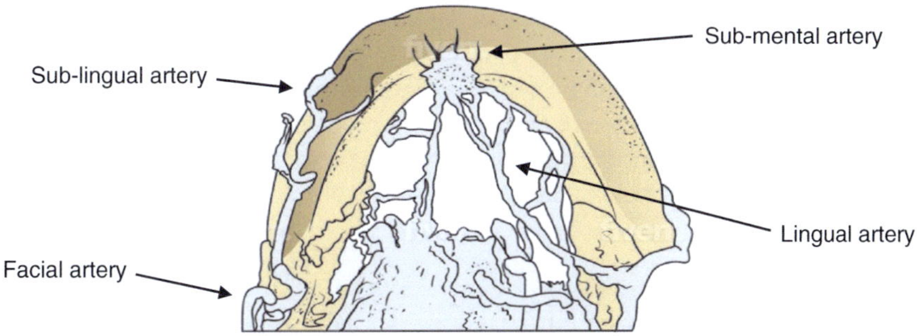


**Fig. 2.4** Diagrammatic illustration of the sub-lingual and sub-mental arteries running along the inferior surface of the anterior mandible

anatomical feature is that both are relatively significant blood vessels within the floor of the mouth and that they frequently anastomose to enter the midline lingual foramen of the mandible [8]. Care must be taken when undertaking osteotomy preparation in the inter-foramina region of the mandible, as haemorrhage leading to upper airway obstruction can occur following transection of the sub-lingual and sub-mental arteries when the lingual cortex or lower boarder of the mandible is perforated during osteotomy preparation. The sequelae of the injury is also compounded as the vessels retract into the floor of the mouth, leading to the formation of a haematoma within the soft-tissue spaces, which can lead to airway compromise. If this occurs, the patient may require surgical intervention in order to stop the haemorrhage and to protect the airway if it is compromised. It is also possible to induce haemorrhaging when elevating the mucogingival flaps lingually if any vessel entering the midline foramen is severed. Therefore, appropriate flap elevation, both buccally and lingually, and visualization of the osteotomy site are required to help avoid iatrogenic hard-tissue perforations. Consideration should also be givemn to changes in hard- and soft-tissue anatomy that occur following tooth loss, and additional imaging may help to plan for safe osteotomy preparation in this region.

*Sub-Mandibular and Sub-Lingual Fossae:* In some patients, there are significant undercuts in the sub-mandibular and sub-lingual regions of the mandible. Whilst these may be present in the dentate patient, their significance can be increased in patients where tooth loss or bony atrophy has occurred. Both fossae form depressions on the medial surface of the mandible inferior to the mylohyoid line and can extend anteriorly to the sub-lingual and sub-mental spaces. They contain the sub-mandibular and sub-lingual glands, respectively [8]. Clinically, the fossa can often be palpated as a shallow depression or undercut on the medial surface of the mandible, lingual and inferior to the alveolar crest.

Ideally, any sub-mandibular or sub-lingual undercuts must be palpated and considered prior to osteotomy preparation, and, if significant, care must be taken not to perforate the lingual bony plate, as this may result in tissue damage and haemorrhage. Sub-mandibular and sub-lingual undercuts can be significant, especially in cases where atrophy exists, and vertical height has been lost. In such cases, the relative height for osteotomy preparation can be significantly reduced when compared to any assessment made using 2D radiographic techniques alone. Direct visualization of the depression can be made intra-operatively; however, if suspected, CBCT imaging will provide you with the most accurate information (Fig. 2.5). Once determined, the site and angulation of any osteotomy preparation and implant placement needs to take into account the position of both the buccal and lingual bone plates, primary or accessory foramina along both aspects of the mandible and any undercuts present.

### 2.2.2 Anatomical Considerations in the Maxilla

*Nasopalatine Foramen:* The nasopalatine or incisive foramen (foramina of Stenson) is located in the midline of the anterior aspect of the maxilla just palatal to the upper central incisors. Within this foramen runs the incisive neurovascular bundle, the anterior branch of the descending palatine vessels and the nasopalatine nerves, which provides sensation to the pre-maxilla and incisor teeth.

The nasopalatine canal and foramen are relatively modest-sized structures (approx. 2–4 mm wide and 8–12 mm in length from the floor of the nose to the alveolus), and although in the majority of the cases they consist of only one canal, on occasions can be significantly larger or consist of multiple canals [9].

An incision made through the incisive papilla does not usually have a detrimental effect on the patient; however, it can occasionally result in paraesthesia of the palatal tissues in the pre-maxillary region, and thus is best avoided. Upon flap reflection, a large incisive canal or the presence of multiple canals maybe an obstacle to implant placement in the incisor region (Fig. 2.6). Following implant placement in the anterior maxilla, persistent or intractable discomfort has been attributed to chronic impingement of the implants on the neurovascular structures in this region. To avoid this problem, either osteotomy preparation and positioning of the implant (if possible) to avoid damage may be required, or ablation and grafting of the canal/s may

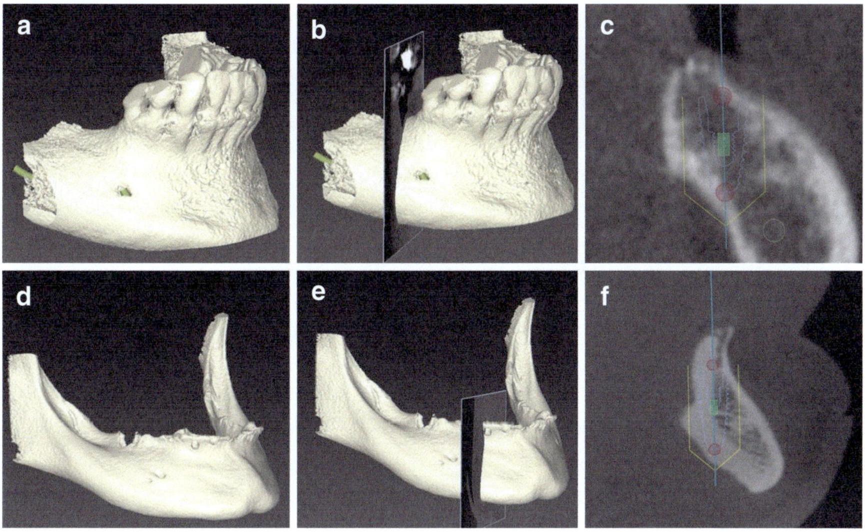


**Fig. 2.5** CBCT images demonstrating the presence of sub-mandibular and sub-lingual fossae and undercuts. When planning implant placement in the mandible, any undercuts on the medial aspect of the lower jaw must be considered. (**a**) 3D reconstructed image of the right posterior mandible from a CBCT scan highlighting the position of the IDN; (**b**) CBCT imaging of the mandible at the site of the lower first molar tooth, where implant placement is planned; (**c**) cross-sectional image at the lower first molar position detailing planned implant position in relation to the alveolar crest and IAN. Note the relative height available is reduced due to the presence of the lingual undercut. (**d**) 3D reconstructed image from a CBCT scan of the right anterior mandible, highlighting the changes in bony anatomy following tooth loss; (**e**) CBCT image of the mandible at the site of the lower canine tooth where implant placement is planned; (**f**) cross-sectional image at the lower canine region detailing planned implant placement in relation to the position of the lower border, sub-lingual undercut and lingual bone plate of the mandible. This demonstrated the difference between the actual and relative heights available for osteotomy preparation and implant placement

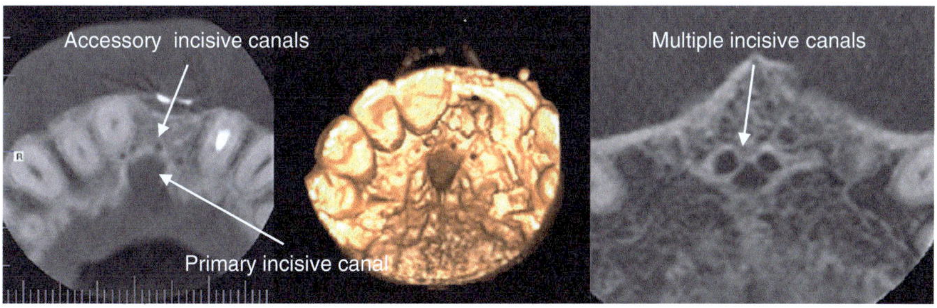


**Fig. 2.6** CBCT images in the axial plane and reconstructed three-dimensional image showing additional foramina lateral and anterior to the primary nasopalatine foramen and three distinct canals at the level of the apices of the adjacent teeth

have to be considered to avoid direct contact with the bundle. Alternatively, if the risk is considered too great, an alternative prosthetic solution may have to be sought.

*Greater Palatine Foramen:* Surgery in the posterior maxilla needs to be undertaken with care. The greater palatine artery and nerve emerge from the respective foramen and traverse the palate anteriorly within the soft tissues of the palatal mucosa. The neurovascular bundle emerges from the palate approximately halfway between the peak of the alveolar crest and midline raphe of the palate. However, the foramen's antero-posterior position along the palate can vary considerably, and its position extends from the third molar (55–85% of cases) to the second molar (1–12% of cases), with the remainder being at some point between the two [10, 11]. Damage to the palatal artery within the soft tissue of the palatal mucosa can be dealt with relatively easily; however, when the damage is close to the foramen, it can present a problem, because the verssel can retract into the greater palatine canal and prevent interventions such as clamping, ligation, or electrocautery. In these instances, a flap design is of utmost importance, and gentle sub-periosteal approach or the precise location of the foramen should be determined prior to flap elevation in the posterior maxilla.

*Maxillary Sinus:* This is the largest of the paranasal sinuses and is bordered by six walls. The anterior wall consists of the facial aspect of the maxilla between the infra-orbital rim and alveolus in the premolar and molar regions of the upper jaw. The superior wall makes up the floor of the orbital and separates the sinus from the orbit. The posterior wall borders the maxillary tuberosity and the pterygo-maxillary region, whilst the medial wall separates the sinus from the nasal passages. The inferior wall consists of the superior aspect of the alveolus and may be encroached upon by the roots of the premolar and molar teeth. The lateral wall extends to and forms the posterior maxillary and zygomatic process, and it is this wall that provides access for the sinus augmentation procedures [12].

Drainage from the sinus is via an opening in the medial maxillary wall, called the ostium, and this is situated on the superior aspect of the medial wall of the maxillary sinus, which communicates from the sinus to the middle meatus of the nose. Given the distance of the ostium from the antral floor, care should be taken not to overfill the sinus when undertaking sinus floor elevation/augmentation procedures, in order to avoid potentially disrupting or blocking the ostium and thus preventing of sinusitis. The sinus floor may extend between the roots of the maxillary premolar and molar teeth and may extend up to 1 cm below the level of the floor of the nasal cavity.

Changes in the hard tissues following tooth loss in the posterior maxilla can vary from individual to individual, and consideration must be given to these changes prior to planning implant placement in this region. Bone loss can occur in both the horizontal and vertical dimensions, and a combination of losses can compound the difficulty when dealing with implant placement in this area (Fig. 2.7). The exact dimensions required for conventional implant placement in the posterior maxilla without the need for augmentation will vary according to the clinician's treatment protocol. However, in recent years, there has been a move away from placing relatively long implants, which required some form of sinus floor augmentation, to a more conservative approach using shorter implants. Given this move, a less invasive

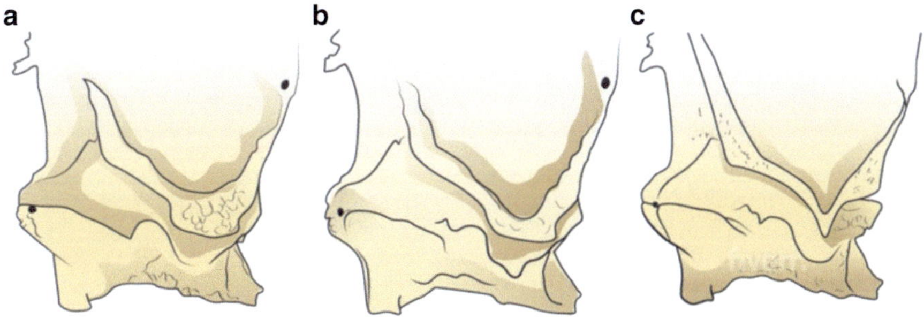

**Fig. 2.7** Diagrammatic illustration showing cross-sections of the posterior maxilla detailing the hard-tissue changes that can occur following tooth loss: (**a**) no bone loss; (**b**) vertical bone loss; (**c**) combination of vertical and horizontal bone loss

approach may be considered, and, therefore, where a residual bone of 6–7 mm width and 8 mm height is present, the latter can be considered without the need for augmentation. Where there is less bone, some form of augmentation will be required to help provide long-term stability for the proposed implants. In cases of extreme maxillary atrophy, alternatives may need to be considered, such block bone grafting, pterygoid or zygomatic implants, or even inter-positional grafting, depending on the clinical scenario.

Sinus floor augmentation can be undertaken either in isolation or simultaneously with implant placement, where conditions are appropriate. Where there is adequate width and 3–4 mm of residual height, simultaneous placement can be undertaken with a high degree of predictability and success. However, where there is less hard tissue, sinus grafting in isolation may be preferred, followed by a period of healing and delayed implant placement (Fig. 2.8). It must be remembered that the objective is to augment the floor of the sinus in order to accommodate the planned size of dental implant to be used for the prosthetic rehabilitation, and not to fill the sinus in its entirety. Care should be taken when undertaking this procedure, as excessive augmentation can lead to soft-tissue changes within the sinus or even direct obstruction of the ostium, which can lead to chronic problems with sinus drainage and symptoms of sinusitis. Augmentation can be undertaken with autologous/autogenous bone, allografts, alloplasts or xenografts and is dependent on clinical indication, personal preference, and patient preference.

Whilst the maxillary sinus may be one continuous structure, septa may often be present, and have been identified in approximately 30% of the sinuses in the premolar and molar areas [13, 14]. Therefore, prior to undertaking sinus floor augmentation procedures, a thorough radiographic evaluation of the anatomy within the sinus should be undertaken in order to anticipate any difficulties that may be faced in terms of root encroachment into the floor of the sinus or position and number of septa present (Fig. 2.9). When negotiating large or multiple septa during such procedures, more than one lateral access hole may need to be created as part of the antral opening in order to prevent tearing of the sinus membrane when reflecting it.

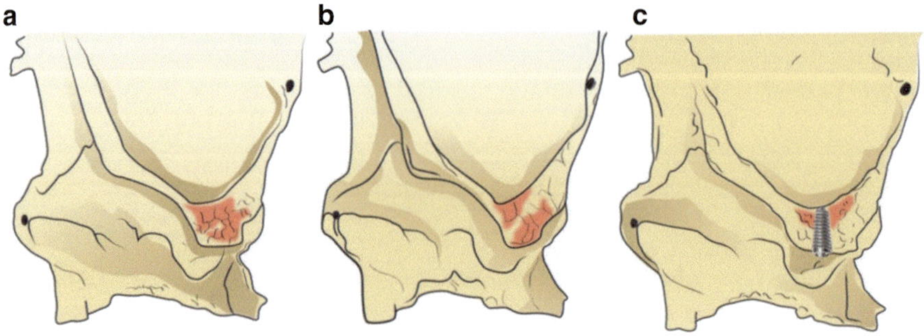


**Fig. 2.8** Diagrammatic illustration detailing cross-sections of the posterior maxilla showing the aims of sinus augmentation: (**a**) sinus floor augmentation to address vertical deficiency; (**b**) augmentation to address a combined deficiency—horizontal and vertical; (**c**) where adequate residual bone is present, simultaneous implant placement with sinus augmentation—note that augmentation is only undertaken to a level to accommodate the size if implant required

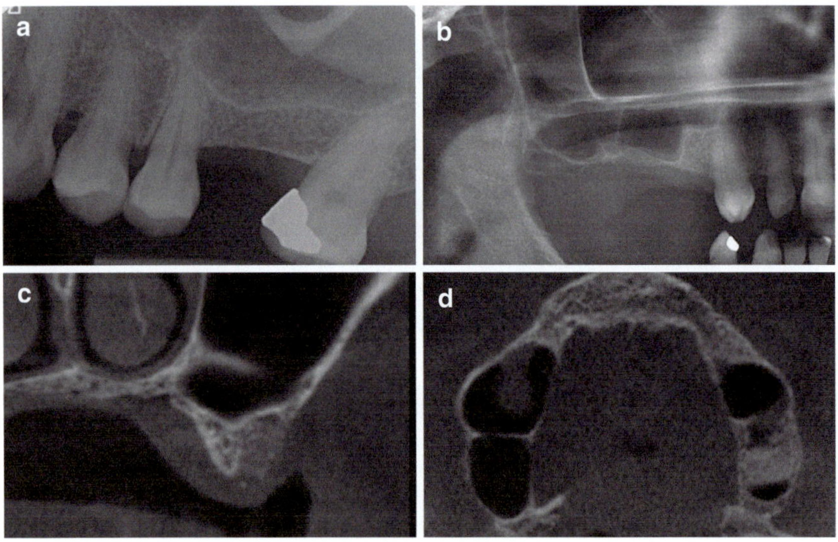


**Fig. 2.9** Radiographic images detailing features when undertaking maxillary sinus procedures. (**a**) Peri-apical radiograph showing anterior extension and vertical bone height with no septa—this may be suitable for simultaneous implant placement; (**b**) half OPT highlighting the vertical bone height and presence of septa on the right maxillary sinus—given the position of the septa, two lateral access holes may need to be undertaken; (**c**) re-formatted CT image (coronal view) of maxilla detailing presence of a horizontal septum; (**d**) re-formatted CT image (coronal view) of maxilla detailing presence of a vertical septum

If a tear in the Schneiderian membrane does occur and it is relatively small, it can be repaired with a small collagen membrane patch. However, when a tear is large and occurs in an area where it is difficult to manage or re-engage the membrane through lateral access hole enlargement then the procedure may have to be aborted, and the site allowed to heal for a period of time before a second attempt is made. The thickness of the sinus membrane can vary considerably, and occasionally may be very thin, thereby making sinus floor augmentation extremely difficult. Conversely, chronic irritation of the sinuses may cause sinus membrane hyperplasia and make the procedure easier than anticipated. However, if the patient suffers from chronic sinus symptoms or has observable sinus pathology, care should be taken when undertaking such procedures, and a second opinion should be sought in relation to such symptoms or pathology.

## References


1. Hatim NA, Al–Rawee RY, Tawfeeq BA. Criteria for selection of Implant cases. Al–Rafidain Dent J. 2006;6(2):161–170.
2. Misch CE. Implant Treatment. Contemporary Implant Dentistry. 1st ed. Mosby Co. St Louis. 1993;4:103–122.
3. Ikeda K, Ho KC, Nowicki BH, Haughton VM. Multiplanar MR and anatomic study of the mandibular canal. AJNR Am J Neuroradiol 1996;17:579–584.
4. Fishel D, Buchner A, Hershkowith A, Kaffe I. Roentgenologic study of the mental foramen. Oral Surg Oral Med Oral Pathol 1976;41:682–686.
5. Ngeow WC, Yuzawati Y. The location of the mental foramen in a selected Malay population. J Oral Sci 2003;45:171–175.
6. Wang TM, Shih C, Liu JC, Kuo KJ. A clinical and anatomical study of the location of the mental foramen in adult Chinese mandibles. Acta Anat [Basel] 1986;126:29–33.
7. Sharawy M. The Companion of Applied Anatomy, vol. 1, 5th ed. Augusta, GA: Medical College of Georgia Printing Service 1995;13.
8. Quirynen M, Mraiwa N, van Steenberghe D, Jacobs R. Morphology and dimensions of the mandibular jaw bone in the interforaminal region in patients requiring implants in the distal areas. Clin Oral Implants Res 2003;14:280–285.
9. Jacobs R, Mraiwa N, Van Cleynenbreugel J, Sanderink G, Schutyser F, et al. The nasopalatine canal revisited using 2D and 3D CT imaging. Dentomaxillofac Radiol 2004;33:396–402.
10. Sujatha N, Manjunath KY, Balasubramanyam V. Variations of the location of the greater palatine foramina in dry human skulls. Indian J Dent Res 2005;16:99–102.
11. Jaffar AA, Hamadah HJ. An analysis of the position of the greater palatine foramen. J Basic Med Sc 2003;3:24–32.
12. Misch CE. The maxillary sinus lift and sinus graft surgery. In: Misch CE, ed. Implant Dentistry, 2nd ed. St Louis: CV Mosby; 1999;469–470.
13. Ulm CW, Solar P, Krennmair G, Matejka M, Watzek G. Incidence and suggested surgical management of septa in sinus-lift procedures. Int J Oral Maxillofac Implants 1995;10:462–465.
14. Mogensen C, Tos M. Quantitative histology of the maxillary sinus. Rhinology 1977;15:129–140.

# Assessment and Treatment Planning

# 3

Shakeel Shahdad

## 3.1 Introduction

A thorough assessment which includes a comprehensive history and clinical examination is essential when planning to replace teeth with dental implants. The majority of the tools and techniques when assessing patients for implants are no different from the ones used in routine dentistry. Therefore, a systematic approach using an assessment form that captures all the necessary information is recommended. A thorough assessment will inform additional special investigations, allowing for appropriate treatment planning and anticipate any complications that may result from the treatment. It can readily inform the clinician of any asymmetry, anomalies, tooth and mucosal colour, texture, ridge deformities and pathologies. Periodontal health is assessed by recording plaque scores, probing the gingival sulcus and measuring any attachment loss. Palpation of the site should be carried out to assess any lumps, bumps and relevant anatomical structures. Percussion of the affected and adjacent teeth should be carried out to aid the diagnosis. Pulp vitality should usually be checked with more than one sensibility test.

Indications for the replacement of teeth with dental implants have been covered in the previous chapter. In summary, a good assessment requires a clinician who has the ability to listen to their patient, respects their wishes and understands their purpose of seeking treatment. Restoration of function, aesthetics and phonetics are the main reasons for our patients seeking treatment with dental implants. It is therefore imperative that the outcome fulfils the patient's expectations.

S. Shahdad (✉)
Oral Rehabilitation & Implantology, Barts and The London School of Medicine and Dentistry, Queen Mary University of London, London, UK

Restorative Dentistry, Royal London Dental Hospital, Barts Health NHS Trust, London, UK
e-mail: s.shahdad@qmul.ac.uk

 
C. Barclay (ed.), *Oral Implantology: Assessment to Maintenance*, BDJ Clinician's Guides, https://doi.org/10.1007/978-3-031-55241-0_3

In edentulous patients, implants can enhance retention and support for a removable prosthesis and are the only modality currently available to provide a fixed solution. Similarly, it is possible to replace single or multiple missing teeth using dental implants without compromising the health of adjacent teeth.

A thorough examination at the initial visit is of fundamental importance to the final outcome. Decisions taken early on will impact on the progression of treatment and ultimately on the end result.

The initial assessment should include:

- Medical history including smoking status
- Social history
- Patients attitude to dentistry
- Lip and smile line
- Extra-oral examination, including mouth opening
- Oral hygiene and periodontal status
- Gingival phenotype and anatomy of soft tissues
- Dental examination (in dentate patients)
- Examination of edentate site and the prosthesis
- Occlusal examination
- Signs of parafunction or bruxism
- Assessment of the implant site
- Special investigations to ascertain:
  - Alveolar bone levels of teeth adjacent to the implant site
  - Anatomy of the alveolar ridge at the implant site
  - Relationship of vital structures to the implant site

## 3.2 Medical History

Ascertaining a thorough medical history is mandatory prior to implant treatment. A systematically obtained medical history should include the general health status, list of medications, allergies and tobacco and alcohol consumption.

Contraindications for implant therapy can be absolute or relative—an absolute contraindication is defined as a medical, psychological or clinical condition due to which implant therapy should not be carried out. On the contrary, a relative contraindication is a condition that may increase the risk of complications, but the benefits of treatment outweigh the risks. An informed consent therefore should always inform the patient of any increased risk for implant failure, intraoperative or postoperative complications. There are very few absolute medical contraindications to placing implants and would include patients with heavily irradiated bone, severe diseases of bone metabolism causing impaired healing, uncontrolled diabetes mellitus, severe immunological conditions or patients who are systemically unwell and cannot undergo the necessary surgery.

The risk of developing osteoradionecrosis has been demonstrated to increase when the accumulated dose of irradiation exceeds 45 Gray. Intensity-modulated radiation therapy may reduce the effective dose of irradiation to the tooth-bearing areas, thereby making implant treatment possible.

The presence of osteoporosis per se does not significantly increase the risk of failure after placing implants. However, osteoporotic patients may be prescribed antiresorptive medication, like bisphosphonates, which may increase the risk for healing, especially after IV bisphosphonate therapy.

Patients receiving antithrombotic treatment warrant caution during and after the surgical procedure. The risk of excessive bleeding during and after standard implant placement should be considered. In general, antithrombotic treatment should not be discontinued since the risk of severe bleeding most often is much lower than the risk of a thromboembolic event. However, the antithrombotic treatment should be adjusted within the therapeutic range after discussion with the patient's physician.

Smoking is not an absolute contraindication for implant therapy, and the impact of smoking on the success of implants has been somewhat controversial with some studies reporting no difference in outcomes between smokers and non-smokers [1], while others have reported a significant negative effect on outcomes except when using more modern implants with particle-blasted, acid-etched or anodic oxidized rough surfaces, especially ultra-hydrophilic implant surfaces [2]. Smokers with a history of periodontitis are at greater risk of developing peri-implantitis [3], and a consensus has now emerged that heavy smoking (over ten cigarettes/day) is associated with higher implant failure. Heavy smokers are considered high-risk, and moderate smokers are considered to be at moderate risk of complications when placing implants [4]. Therefore, the patient should be informed about the increased risk of implant loss and peri-implant disease, and complete smoking cessation, or at least a reduction the in number of cigarettes, should be encouraged.

Alcohol consumption may not directly influence the implant success and survival, but the main problem is related to compounding factors such as liver disease and malnutrition. Furthermore, alcohol abuse may present with poor oral hygiene and compliance issues.

## 3.3 Social History

Implant therapy is potentially complex, and it is prudent to ascertain if patients are able to commit to the treatment in terms of time, surgical side effects and its impact on their life style or work commitments.

## 3.4 Patients' Expectations and Attitude to Dentistry

Is the treatment the patient wants realistically achievable, and can it be achieved in the time frame the patient wants? Aesthetics are often the main driver of motivation for patients to seek treatment and it is therefore imperative that the outcome fulfils the patient's expectations. Is the expected treatment realistic and achievable within the timeframe? Aesthetics are subjective, and negotiating patient expectations in accordance with what can be realistically and predictably achieved will avoid later disagreements. Implants, when planned, inserted and prosthetically restored appropriately, should be able to achieve an excellent aesthetic outcome.

## 3.5 Lip and Smile Line

Patients will show different proportions of their anterior dento-alveolar process on full smile. The smile can be divided into three categories. In a low smile line, less than 75% of the incisal length is exposed and the gingival margins or tips of the papillae of their maxillary teeth are not visible, and, therefore, the contour of the gingivae around the implant-retained restoration is less critical than in patients with a high lip line (Fig. 3.1a). In a high smile line, the entire clinical crown with surrounding gingival tissues is exposed (Fig. 3.1b), and, therefore, the level of precision required in handling the soft-tissue profile around implants is less forgiving and will require efforts to maintain peri-implant tissue support throughout the various phases of treatment. A patient with an average smile line reveals the interproximal papilla (Fig. 3.1c).

## 3.6 Extra-oral Examination Including Mouth Opening

Extra-oral examination includes assessment of the temporomandibular joints, muscles of mastication and regional lymph nodes. Pain or temporomandibular joint dysfunction requires further evaluation prior to complex implant therapy.

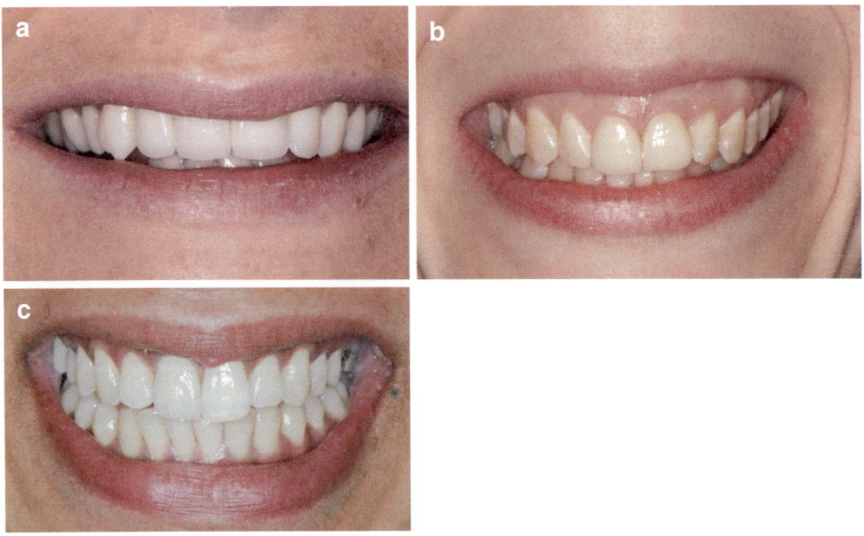

**Fig. 3.1** (**a**) Low smile line. (**b**) High smile line. (**c**) Average smile line

Mouth opening needs to be sufficient to accommodate the hand-piece and drills when placing an implant and, therefore, should be assessed and recorded at consultation.

## 3.7 Oral Hygiene and Periodontal Status

A basic periodontal examination is mandatory to ascertain the presence or absence of periodontal disease and any active periodontal disease should be treated before embarking on implant therapy. Periodontitis results in resorption of the alveolar bone around the teeth, and, as a consequence, the alveolar bone height is reduced and may limit the available bone height, particularly in the vicinity of the maxillary sinus and the inferior dental canal (Fig. 3.2a). Periodontitis also causes gingival recession, including the interdental papilla. Patients should be adequately warned that replacement with implants is unlikely to restore the papillae (Fig. 3.2b).

The patient compliance and their ability to perform oral hygiene procedures should be ascertained before implant treatment begins. Evidence suggests that patients with history of periodontal disease, poor oral hygiene and microbial biofilms are at greater risk of peri-implant infections, implant loss and other complications than disease-free individuals [3, 5].

## 3.8 Gingival Phenotype and Anatomy of Soft Tissues

Patients have different gingival tissues in terms of appearance, contour and thickness [6]. These are referred to as gingival phenotypes and are broadly categorized as either thin, medium or thick.

Thick phenotypes are considered to be fibrous in appearance with flat or minimal scalloping and a wide band of keratinized mucosa (Fig. 3.3a). On the contrary, the thin phenotype is identified with thin mucosa, high scalloped margins and a narrow

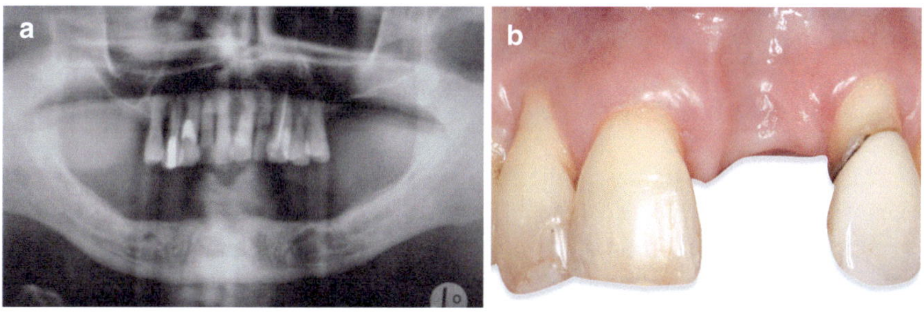


**Fig. 3.2** (**a**) OPG of a patient with periodontitis showing alveolar ridge resorption in maxilla and mandible with insufficient bone for placement of implants in posterior maxilla and mandible. (**b**) Attachment loss due to periodontitis has resulted in loss of interdental bone as well, which will influence the aesthetic outcome after restoration of the missing tooth with dental implant

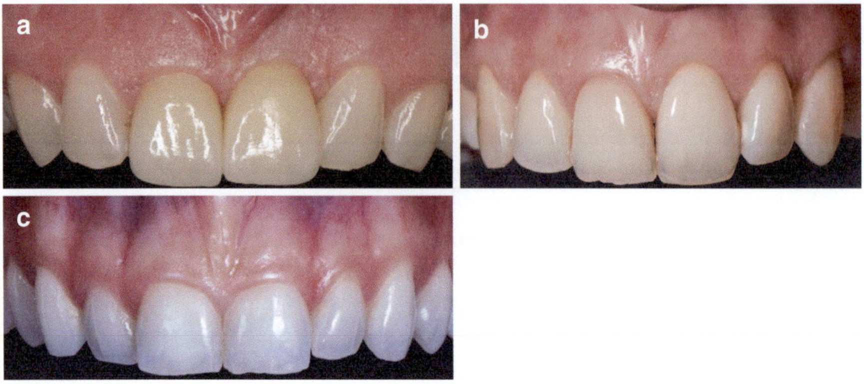


**Fig. 3.3** (**a**) Thick phenotype. (**b**) Thin phenotype. (**c**) Medium phenotype

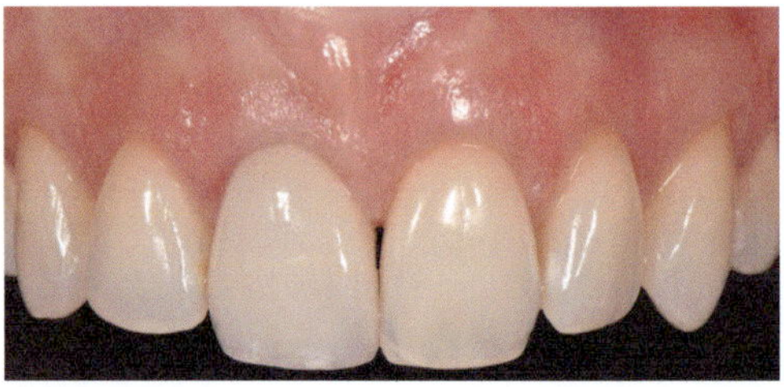

**Fig. 3.4** UR1 has been replaced in a patient with thin phenotype with excellent aesthetic outcome

band of keratinized mucosa (Fig. 3.3b). The medium phenotype displays some characteristics of the thick phenotype (thick attached gingival tissues) and thin phenotype (long, thin and blunted dental papillae) (Fig. 3.3c).

There is a correlation between the phenotype and the thickness of the labial bone of the alveolar socket, with thin phenotype tending to have a thin labial bone compared to medium or thick phenotypes. A thin phenotype is prone to gingival recession [7]. A thick phenotype is considered to be low-risk and resistant to recession around implants, shows less papilla loss and may also mask the colour of the implant and metallic implant abutment [8]. However, when correctly executed, excellent aesthetic outcomes can be achieved in thin gingival cases (Fig. 3.4).

The gingival phenotype is assessed by using a periodontal probe in the gingival crevice; a probe that shines through the gingiva signifies a thin phenotype (Fig. 3.5) [9].

Additionally, soft tissues in the implant site should be examined for any deficiency regarding volume and quantity. Soft-tissue deficiency usually correlates with an underlying hard-tissue deficiency, and augmentation of both hard and soft tissues may have to be considered for successful outcome.

It is desirable for implants to be surrounded by sufficient amounts of keratinized tissue. There is no evidence that increasing the width of keratinized tissue improves the prognosis of implants, although increased amounts of plaque and inflammation are found around implants with less than 2-mm width of keratinized mucosa.

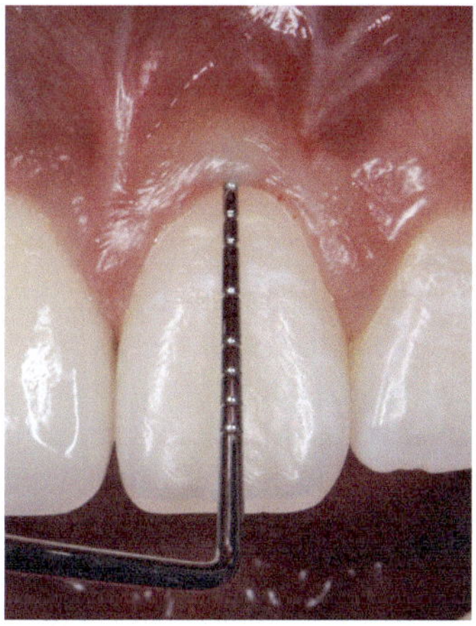

**Fig. 3.5** Assessment of gingival phenotype using a periodontal probe

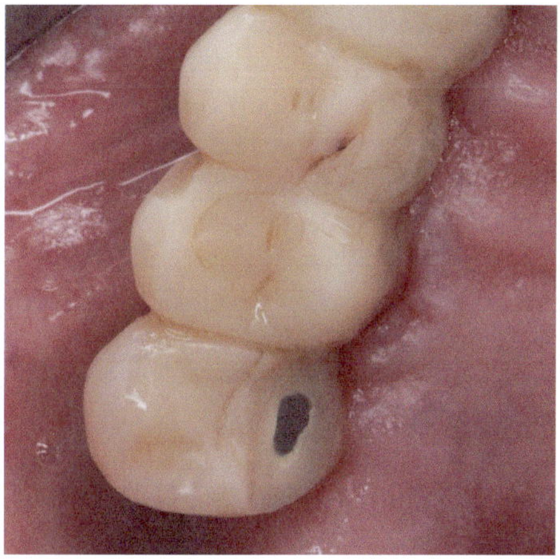

**Fig. 3.6** Ceramic delamination (chipping) in a patient with full-arch metal–ceramic implant-fixed bridge is one of the common complications especially in patients with a history of bruxism

## 3.9 Signs of Parafunction or Bruxism

Parafunction remains a controversial issue, as there is no evidence that directly correlates bruxism to implant failure [10], although implants will be under increased occlusal loading, and especially non-axial loading of implants can lead to increased mechanical failures such as screw loosening, screw and abutment fracture as well as technical complications such as prosthesis fracture or chipping of ceramic (Fig. 3.6) [11, 12]. An occlusal splint is recommended for patients with parafunctional habits to minimize the aforementioned complications.

## 3.10 Dental Examination (in Dentate Patients)

Implant therapy should be avoided in patients with ongoing active dental disease, even though caries does not directly influence the success rates of implants. A thorough dental examination will reveal evidence of any caries, pulpal or periapical disease, and the extent of existing restorations that would influence the long-term prognosis of the remaining dentition. Any teeth with guarded prognosis should be considered so that the oral environment is rendered disease-free and stable before embarking on implant therapy. At the least, the treatment plan should account for their failure in future, and dismantling of restorations might be necessary to establish prognosis of individual teeth, especially the ones within the vicinity of the planned implant restoration.

There are various dental factors that may influence implant therapy and include the age of the patient, the reason for tooth loss and previous implant history or experience. Information about previous implant history provides valuable insight into the patient's compliance, expectations and ability to tolerate implant treatment.

Implants should not be placed in children and adolescents until craniofacial growth has reached their full skeletal maturity. Dental implants behave like ankylosed teeth, and in a growing jaw, they do not erupt along with the surrounding jawbone. The surrounding alveolar bone remains under-developed, and the implant restoration can become infra-occluded if placed too early (Fig. 3.7a, b).

Older age is usually not a contraindication or a risk factor for implant loss. However, age should be considered in conjunction with other medical factors such as compromised health, because of which the patient may not tolerate the surgery, or protracted treatment, and compliance with maintenance.

Implants should be not placed in infected sites and when assessing the site, the periapical status of the neighbouring teeth should also be examined to avoid future complications. A chronic endodontic infection will inevitably result in bone resorption in the periapical area, which would influence implant treatment due to deficient bone volume (Fig. 3.8a–c). Any residual pathology or inflammation may also adversely affect the outcome due to failure of implant osseointegration. Bone resorption is likely to be worse if an endodontic surgery has been carried out previously. The resultant bone deficiency will require a bone graft at the time of implant placement.

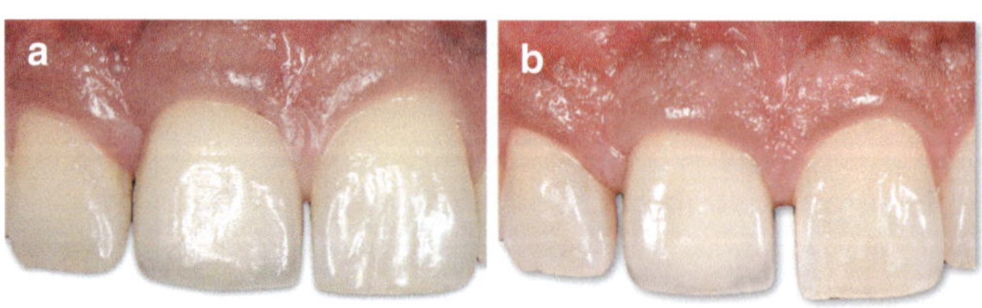


**Fig. 3.7** (**a**) Definitive implant crown fit at the age of 19 years. (**b**) Same crown 13 y later—note the continuing maxillary alveolar growth with an incisal step and diastema developing between the adjacent teeth

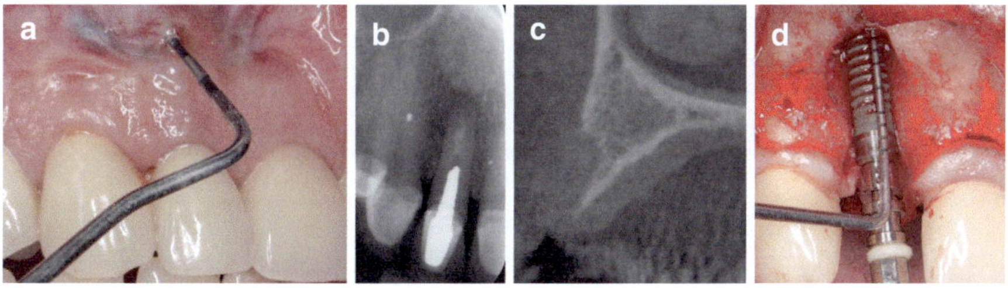


**Fig. 3.8** (**a** and **b**) UR2 with a post and core crown presenting with a history of two previous apical surgeries (amalgam retrograde followed by MTA). Amalgam tattooing of the mucosa and a persistently draining apical sinus are present. (**c**) CBCT scan taken 5 weeks after extraction confirms complete resorption of the facial bone plate. (**d**) Implant is placed 6 weeks after extraction, and the anticipated bone dehiscence will require simultaneous bone grafting utilizing the guided bone regeneration (GBR) technique

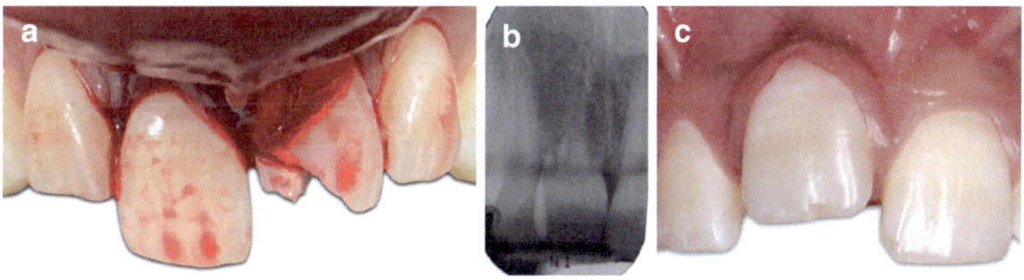


**Fig. 3.9** (**a**) Immediate dento-alveolar trauma in UR1 and enamel-dentine fracture in UL1. (**b**) Previously avulsed and re-implanted tooth now showing signs on non-infected replacement resorption. (**c**) Clinical picture of the tooth in Fig. 3.9b showing the effects of avulsion resulting in infraocclusion of UR1

Dento-alveolar trauma may result in substantial damage to the teeth and alveolar ridge (Fig. 3.9a), requiring bone augmentation for successful implant therapy. Previously avulsed teeth may also undergo ankylosis with subsequent replacement resorption, internal and external inflammatory resorption and cervical root resorption (Fig. 3.9b). Ankylosis of a re-implanted tooth in a child usually results in infraocclusion, thereby complicating the clinical situation (Fig. 3.9c).

Congenitally missing teeth adversely affect the development of the alveolar process, and these patients most often have a significant alveolar bone deficiency, thereby necessitating bone augmentation procedures, either staged or simultaneously at the time of implant placement (Fig. 3.10a–c). Hypodontia patients often have concomitantly malpositioned and/or malformed teeth. It is imperative that these patients are managed by a multidisciplinary team of specialists. This includes orthodontic treatment to reposition teeth, paediatric and restorative teams to manage the dental problems.

Ectopic teeth, primarily maxillary canines, often pose a clinical problem and may not be amenable to orthodontic alignment. This decision should be taken in collaboration with an orthodontist. The position of an ectopic tooth might interfere with the proposed position of a dental implant, and its surgical extraction might be necessary, resulting in a significant alveolar bone defect.

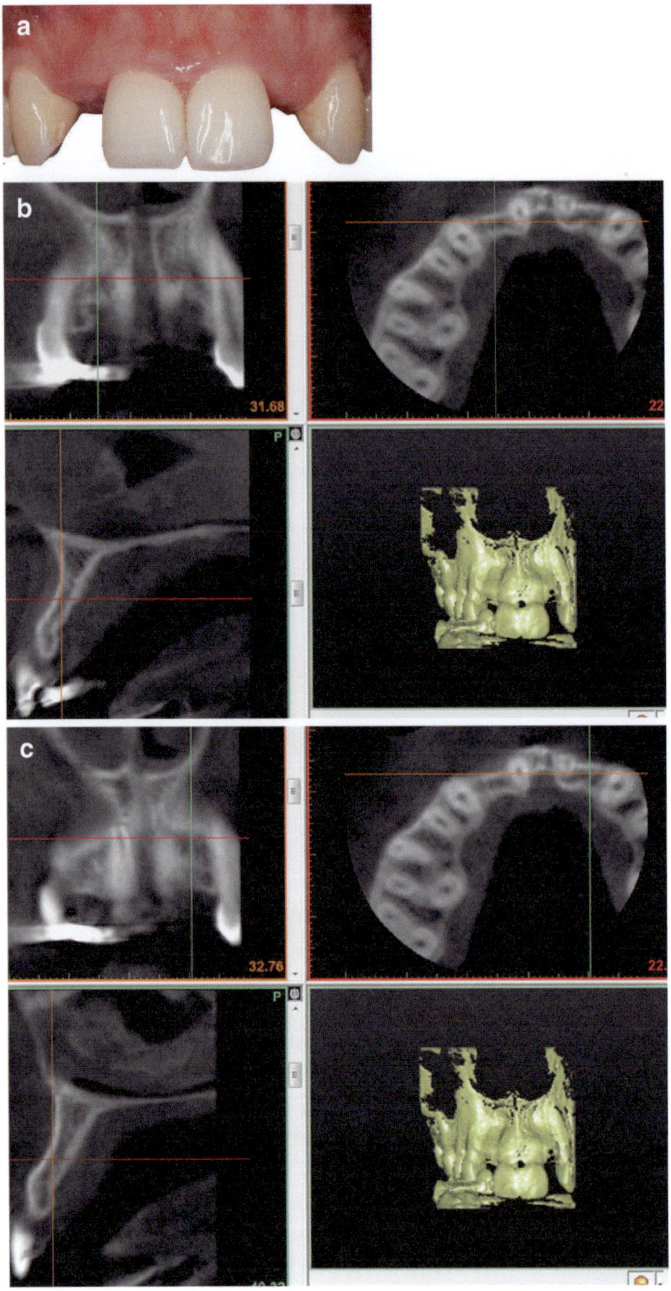

**Fig. 3.10** (**a**) Congenitally missing maxillary lateral incisors. (**b** and **c**) CBCT imaging reveals significantly atrophied lateral incisor sites

## 3.11 Examination of Edentate Site and the Prosthesis

Examination of Edentate Site and the Prosthesis: Edentulous patients are often referred to as "oral cripples" and implants can provide significant improvement in the overall quality of life. In 2002, the McGill Consensus Statement emphasised that the minimum standard of care for edentulous mandibles is a two-implant overdenture as it significantly improves the stability compared to traditional dentures, enhancing patient satisfaction and oral function [13]. This was followed by the York Consensus in 2009, highlighting the need for individualised treatment planning, recognising that while fixed full-arch prostheses might provide superior aesthetics and function, they require careful patient selection and a higher initial investment [14].

When evaluating the edentate site for prosthetic options, clinicians must decide between opting for an implant-retained overdenture or a fixed full-arch prosthesis. This choice significantly impacts functional outcomes and patient satisfaction. Key factors influencing this decision include:

- Anatomical Considerations: The quantity of bone present at the edentate site dictates the type of prosthesis that can be supported. Adequate bone volume across the arch where implants are to be placed is necessary for a fixed prosthesis. In contrast, mandibular overdentures only require two implants in the inter-canine area and very rarely, a clinical situation arises where two implants cannot be accommodated.
- Aesthetic Considerations: Edentulous patients with severe alveolar ridge resorption lack lip support and often a denture flange is required to provide the necessary support for the lip and ensuring the teeth are in the correct position (Fig. 3.11a–j). Therefore, in such clinical situations, implant-retained removable overdenture is the best option even though bone volume to accommodate implant might be available.
- Functional Needs: Fixed prostheses generally offer superior functional outcomes compared to overdentures, although research does not support this perception. However, the patient's expectations and ability to maintain oral hygiene are crucial factors. A fixed prosthesis requires excellent hygiene maintenance, which might be challenging for some patients.
- Patient's Health Status: Systemic health factors like dexterity and cognitive ability can influence the choice. For patients with limited manual dexterity or cognitive issues, an overdenture might be preferable due to easier maintenance and handling.
- Economic Factors: The cost differences between the two options can be significant. Implant-retained overdentures are generally less expensive and require fewer implants, which might be a decisive factor for many patients.
- Long-term Maintenance: Consideration of the long-term durability and maintenance requirements is essential. Fixed prostheses, while offering a more natural function, may require more complex and costly maintenance compared to overdentures.

These guidelines suggest that the choice between an implant-retained overdenture and a fixed full arch should be tailored to the individual's specific needs, medical condition, and economic capacity. By carefully considering these factors, clinicians can ensure optimal outcomes that align with the patient's lifestyle and expectations.

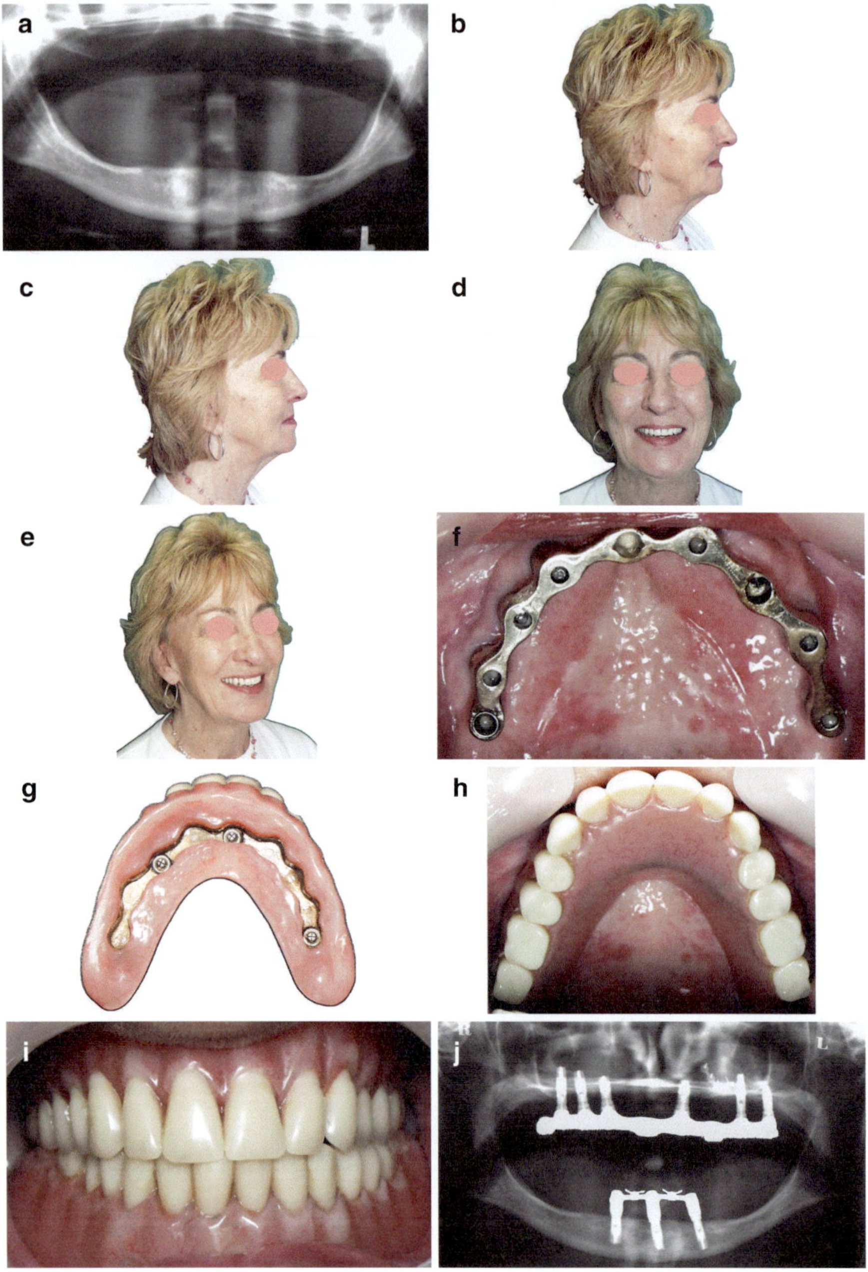

## 3.12 Assessment of the Implant Site

The site-specific assessments include the restorative space, anatomical factors and hard and soft tissues, including any pathoses in the area. A prosthodontically driven site assessment and treatment planning underpin the overall treatment success. Assessment of the restorative space and its characteristics makes it possible to determine any space limitations, anticipate treatment complexity and assess any risk of complications.

The examination should assess whether the three-dimensional space is adequate for the prosthetic tooth replacement. The examination should include the mesio-distal space (Fig. 3.11a–d), the bucco-lingual space (Fig. 3.12), the interocclusal space (Fig. 3.13a–c) and the interradicular space (Fig. 3.14).

The defined minimum mesio-distal space between adjacent teeth should be available to replace a tooth with an optimally sized prosthetic reconstruction, and the size of the tooth will determine the ideal diameter of the planned implant. For example, a lateral incisor should be replaced with a narrower-diameter implant than a molar. A minimum distance of 1.5 mm between the implant and the adjacent tooth should be maintained to prevent complications and damage to the tooth and its root. If an implant is placed too close to an adjacent tooth, the interdental bone will resorb, and with it the papilla, resulting in an un-aesthetic black triangle. A distance of 1.5 mm or greater is recommended between an implant and an adjacent tooth. When replacing multiple teeth, mesio-distal space will dictate the size of teeth to be replaced, which will determine the number and optimal diameters of the implants to be placed. A minimum distance of 3 mm between adjacent implants has been shown to maintain the interimplant bone crest and the associated papilla [15–17]. However, we would recommed a 4mm inter-implant distance to better control inter-implant soft tissue (papilla).

The interocclusal space (space from the crestal mucosa of the implant site to the opposing dentition) should also be measured. This requires assessment of the overall volume of space with the teeth in occlusion. Apart from assessing overjet and overbite, any overeruption of opposing teeth should be carefully assessed. This static and dynamic relationship will influence whether the prosthesis will be

**Fig. 3.11** (**a**) Pre-operative panoramic radiograph of an edentulous patient requesting a maxillary and mandibular fixed implant prosthesis (**b**) 3.11b – Side profile of the patient without any prosthesis shows the collapse of the maxillary lip due to severe anterior maxillary alveolar resorption and the resultant lack of lip support (**c**) Side profile with maxillary and mandibular denture try-in showing adequate lip support and optimal facial profile. Such a clinical assessment confirms the need for a labial flange in the maxillary denture to achieve the ideal aesthetic outcome (**d**, **e**) Pleasing aesthetic outcome with the proposed tooth set-up (**f**) Six maxillary implants placed connected with a cast gold bar incorporating milled parallel walls and overdenture attachments (**g**, **h**, **i**) Denture converted to a removable prosthesis with a cast oversleeve with additional attachments. In essence, this results in a removable prosthesis with significantly high retention and stability and reduced palatal coverage whilst providing a flange and an ability to set teeth in an ideal position for optimal lip and cheek support for aesthetics (**j**) Post-operative panoramic radiograph showing maxillary and mandibular implants

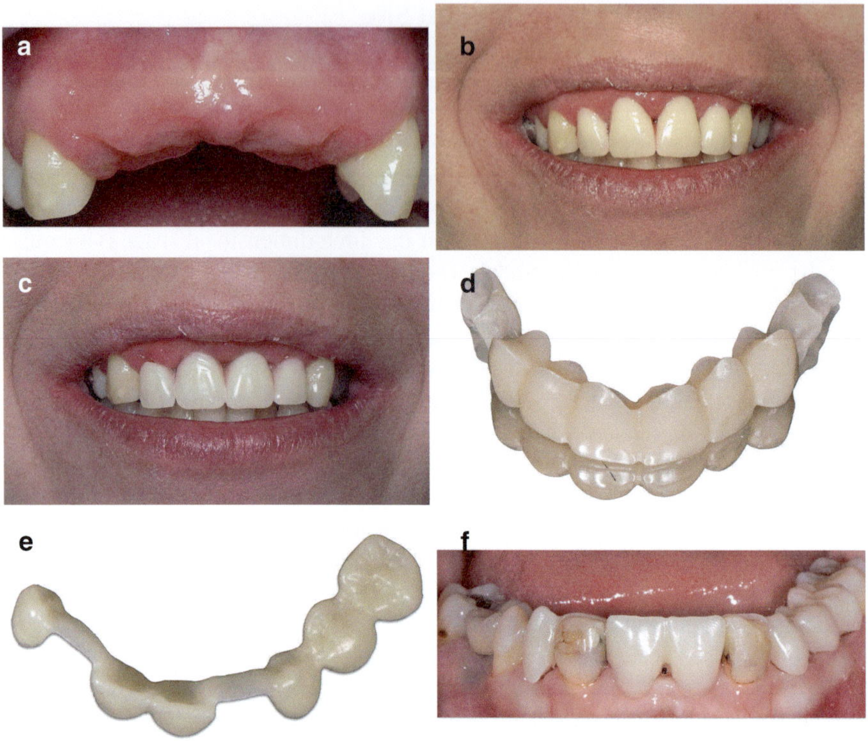

**Fig. 3.12** (**a**, **b**, **c**) Diagnostic planning for replacement of maxillary incisors. Two different tooth size plans allow for the visualisation of the proposed treatment. Maxillary incisor proportion in 3.12b resulted in a better aesthetic outcome in relation to patients' natural dentition. Finalising the zenith of proposed implant positions during planning is critical to optimise implant depth according to the diagnostic wax-up (**d**, **e**) With advances in digital workflows, traditional diagnostic plans using denture teeth and wax can be replaced with milled or 3d printed prosthetic try-ins (**f**) The milled PMMA prototype can be tried in the mouth (**g**) stl file of the diagnostic plan is imported to an implant planning software to allow for ideal prosthetically guided implant position and designing of the surgical guide (**h**, **i**) Fully guided surgical protocol to facilitate optimal implant positioning based on the virtual implant plan (**j**) Implants placed through the surgical guide. A fully guided implant protocol can benefit the patient and the clinician. However, it should be noted that guided surgery is not entirely accurate, and clinical experience is essential to recognise its limitations

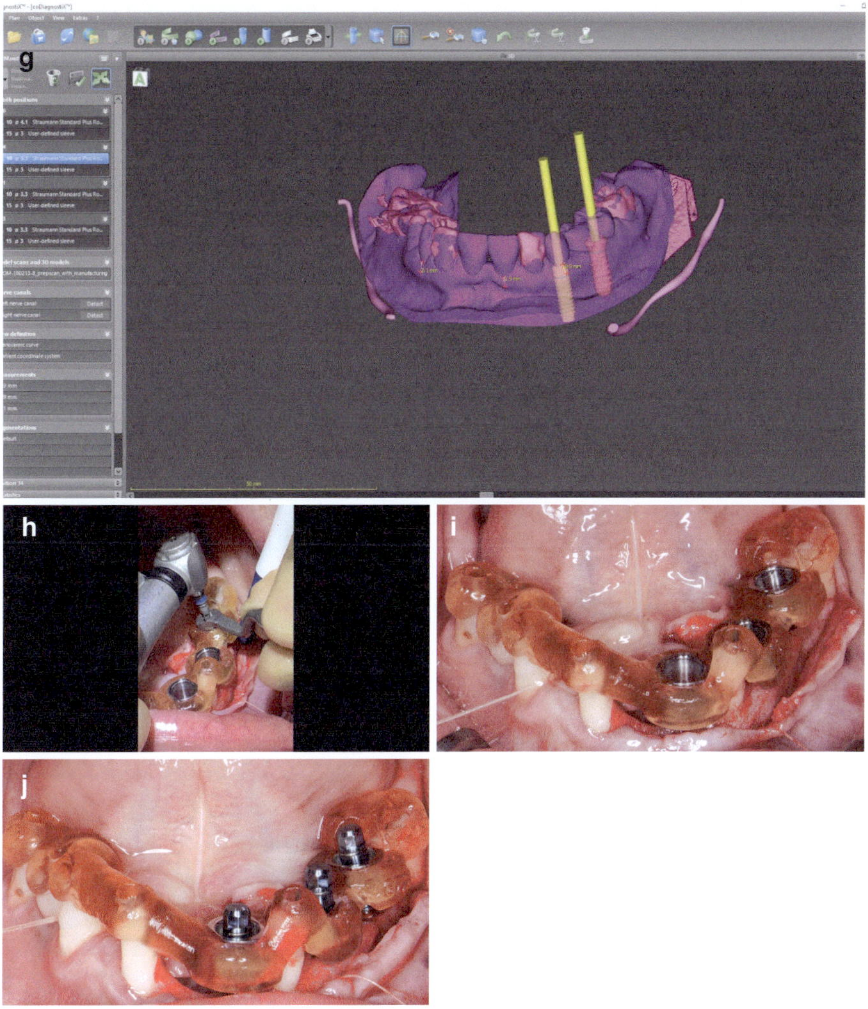


**Fig. 3.12** (continued)

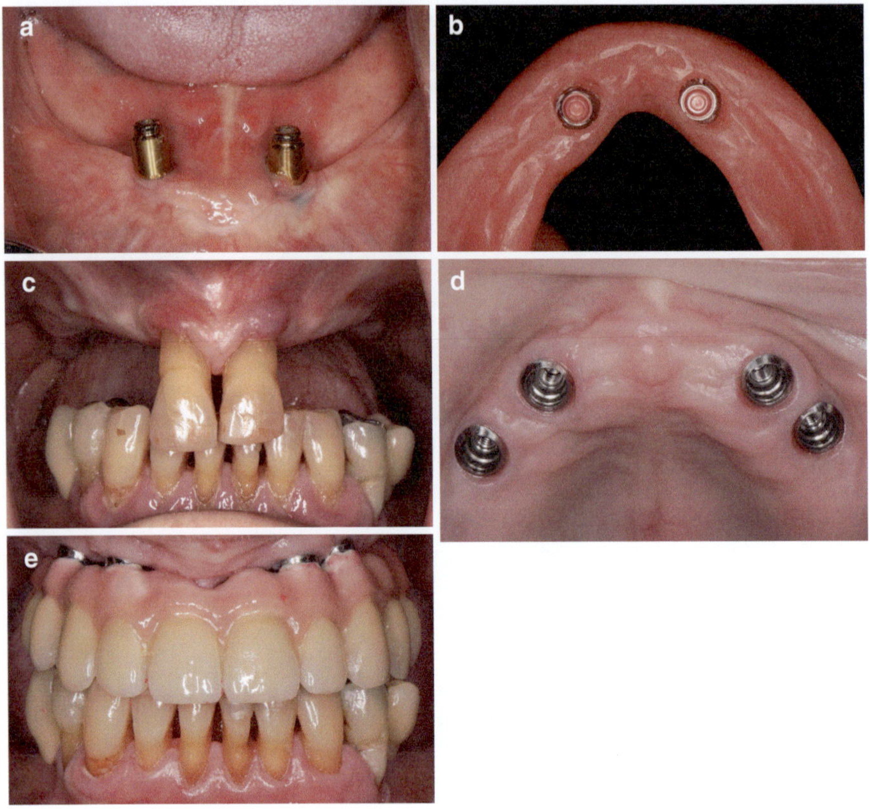

**Fig. 3.13** (**a**) Two mandibular intra-foraminal implants with overdenture abutments (**b**) Female housing in the denture to help enhance denture retention (**c**) Example of a patient with severe xerostomia secondary to Sjogren's syndrome. Removable dentures in xerostomia patients can be uncomfortable and discomfort even if retention were enhanced with the aid of dental implants (**d**, **e**) A fixed implant prosthesis is better tolerated by patients with xerostomia or other mucosal conditions where rubbing from a removable prosthesis might be painful (**f**) Milled bar with incorporated retentive elements to aid implant stabilised removable prosthesis in a patient with severe gag reflex. This is virtually a removable bridge with excellent retention and stability (**g**, **h**) Screw retained maxillary fixed implant prosthesis on six implants

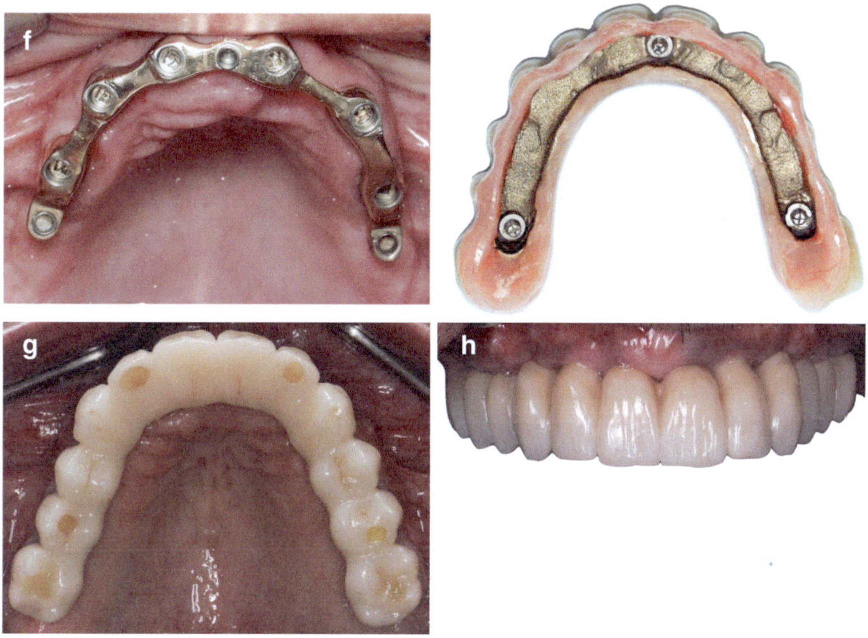


**Fig. 3.13** (continued)

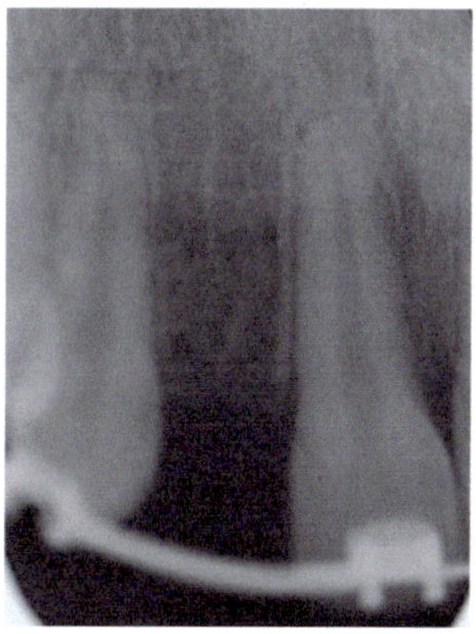

**Fig. 3.14** Assessment of interradicular space can be performed with a plain film intraoral peri-apical radiograph

screw- or cement-retained (Fig. 3.13b). An interocclusal space of at least 4 mm is desirable for a straightforward implant restoration. Deep anterior overbite might be the only clinical situation where cement-retained restoration is preferred due to the limited space to accommodate the screw channel.

In the posterior region, a limited interocclusal space may represent an absolute contraindication for implant therapy. From a prosthetic point of view, an implant restoration requires enough space for the abutment and the crown. Fig. 3.13c demonstrates a case of an extreme example where the mandibular molars have significantly over-erupted with barely any space available for replacement of the maxillary teeth.

A minimum interradicular space between adjacent teeth is necessary to prevent damage to the periodontal ligament and roots of the adjacent teeth from implants. Orthodontic treatment may be indicated to create sufficient space for an implant (Fig. 3.14), or an alternative non-implant restoration should be offered to the patient.

Examinations, particularly in posterior regions of the jaw, can be facilitated with accurately articulated casts (Fig. 3.15a, b).

A diagnostic tooth set-up or wax-up, particularly when multiple teeth are to be replaced is essential for thorough planning (Fig. 3.16a, b).

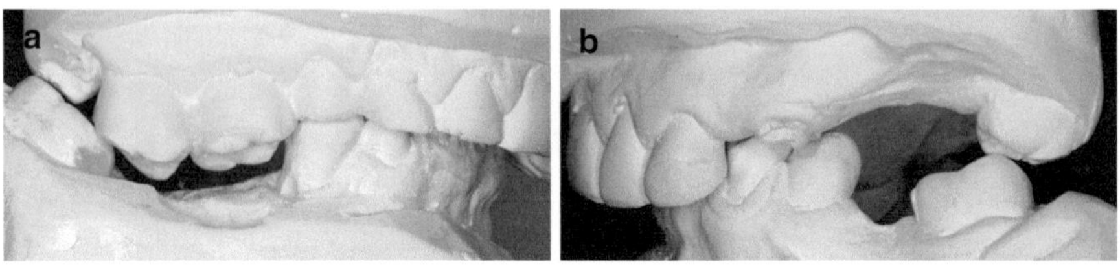


**Fig. 3.15** (**a** and **b**) Accurately articulated study models can allow for better assessment of intricate occlusal relationship and interferences in a case like this with undesirable over-eruption of teeth

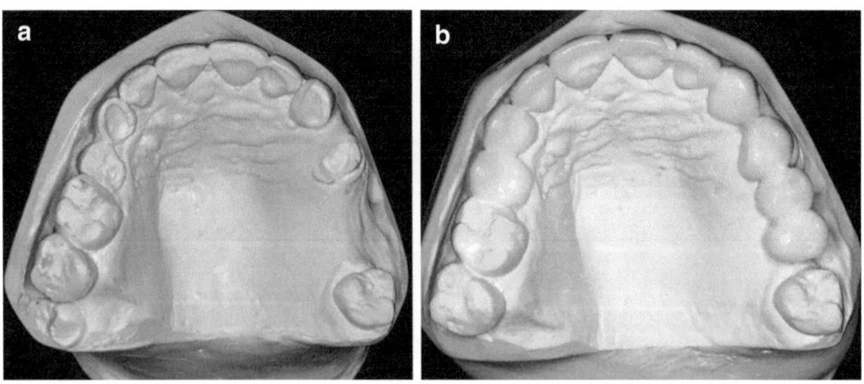


**Fig. 3.16** (**a** and **b**) Planning for replacement of missing teeth in UL quadrant is planned with diagnostic wax-up

### 3.12.1 Anatomy of the Alveolar Ridge at the Implant Site

A critical aspect of planning is careful examination of the alveolar ridge and overlying soft tissues (Fig. 3.17a, b). Such examinations will inform treatment decisions, such as carrying out bone or soft-tissue grafting procedures as part of implant therapy.

Implants can be placed in fresh extraction sockets (immediate placement, Type I), following a 6–8 week period of healing (Type II) or many months after the natural tooth was lost (Types III and IV) [18]. Each of these scenarios is slightly different and requires a different form of assessment. Appropriate radiographs or scans are, of course, mandatory prior to any surgical intervention. If the implant is to be placed immediately following extraction, the socket anatomy can be explored directly with a probe at the time of surgery (Fig. 3.18).

If the implant is to be placed more than 4 months following extraction, approximately 50% of the width of the labial plate will have been lost, with 30% of the palatal bony wall similarly affected [19]. Type II placement is preferred in the aesthetic zone in order to achieve the most optimal aesthetics.

Cone beam CT scanning now makes it possible to measure the width of the residual ridge using computer software [20].

In the aesthetic zone, the ideal tooth position must be determined prior to any surgery. The implant position then follows the ideal position of the crown.

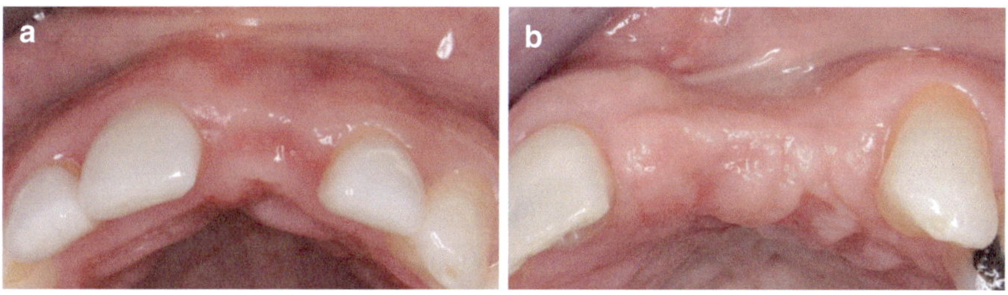

**Fig. 3.17** (**a**) Clinical situation with adequate bone volume for placement of implant, whereas (**b**) shows significant alveolar ridge width atrophy, and a staged augmentation with a block bone graft is very likely required

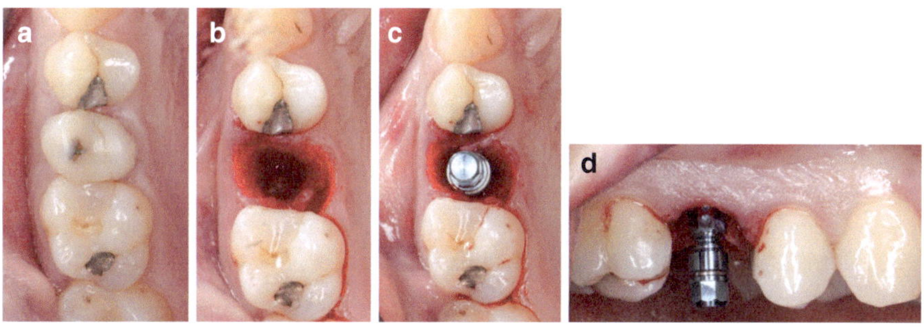

**Fig. 3.18** (**a**) An example of Immediate (Type 1) implant placement of UR5, (**b**) extraction socket is explored and any graulation tissue is removed (**c**, **d**) implant position check in three dimensions

### 3.12.2 Relationship of Vital Structures to the Implant Site

The location of vital structures can limit the dimensions of implants and consequently may render implants an unfeasible treatment option. These include the incisive foramen and the nasopalatine canal, the nose, the maxillary sinus, the inferior dental canal, the mental foramen, the inferior border of the mandible and the lingual concavity.

After the loss of teeth, maxillary sinus pneumatization is commonly noticed, and the floor of the sinus may drop down so that there is insufficient bone height left for an implant. Therefore, a bone augmentation inside the maxillary sinus may be necessary in which a lateral window allows entry into the sinus and a bone substitute is placed after careful elevation of the sinus membrane to increase the height of the alveolar ridge.

In the anterior maxilla, the floor of the nose is the limiting anatomical factor. Unlike in the maxillary sinus, bone augmentation to increase the ridge height at the nasal floor is complex and very rarely recommended.

The mental foramen is an important landmark. The position of the foramen should be accurately identified to prevent damage to the neurovascular bundle, which exits the foramen. CBCT imaging is indicated to most accurately locate and plan dental implant selection and positioning.

Distal to the mental foramen, the inferior alveolar canal should be identified to prevent damage to the neurovascular bundle. A distance of at least 2 mm from the canal is recommended to avoid damage to the nerve.

In a resorbed or severely resorbed mandible, the inferior border of the mandible limits the implant length.

In the posterior mandible, a lingual concavity might be present, which is best assessed on a CBCT. It is important to identify this, since perforations of the lingual cortex during osteotomy can result in sublingual haemorrhage, causing airway obstruction and potential death.

## 3.13 Special Investigations

After a thorough clinical examination, appropriate radiographs should be considered to gain additional information. Intraoral radiographs, dental panoramic or low-dose cone beam computed tomograms are most appropriate.

The intraoral examination is often inadequate for full assessment and planning, and articulated study casts are required for a thorough analysis. A diagnostic wax-up is an invaluable aid when assessing and planning replacement of teeth. In some cases, a denture tooth set-up is more appropriate. A diagnostic wax-up can be visually shown to a patient, whereas a denture tooth set-up can also be tried inside the mouth, allowing both patient and clinician a much better perspective of the planned treatment (Fig 3.12a–c). Recent advances in digital technology and the increasing availability of intra-oral scanners and CAD-CAM have added an entirely new dimension to implant dentistry. Together with virtual implant planning software, prosthetic and implant planning allow for safe and efficient treatment protocols, especially when combined with guided implant surgery (Fig 3.12d–j).

## 3.14 Treatment Planning Decisions

One of the main indications for implant therapy is to restore function. Missing teeth need replacement if the individual cannot masticate efficiently or comfortably.

Implants can also offer significant improvement regarding aesthetics and phonetics. In edentulous patients, they may improve retention and support of removable dental prostheses. With implants it is possible to provide a fixed prosthesis to replace single or multiple missing teeth. Often, it is the patients' desire to replace their missing teeth with a fixed prosthesis and without jeopardizing the long-term health and survival of potential adjacent abutment teeth, which would serve as abutments for conventional fixed dental prosthesis. Preparing teeth as abutments leads to irreversible destruction of tooth tissue, with a potential loss of vitality and compromised long-term health. In contrast, implants allow replacement of missing teeth without compromising the health of adjacent teeth.

Implants, when planned, inserted and prosthetically restored appropriately, should be able to achieve an excellent aesthetic and functional outcome. Aesthetics are often the main driver of motivation for patients to seek treatment. It is therefore imperative that the outcome fulfils the patient's expectations.

Patients struggling with the retention of their maxillary or mandibular conventional removable dental prosthesis may also struggle with speech. Enhancing retention by offering an implant-supported prosthesis can improve the phonetics as well.

Implants are indicated when enhancement of retention and support for a removable dental prosthesis is desirable. Particularly in severely resorbed mandibles, prostheses can cause pain due to excessive movements during function. Implant-retained prostheses on two implants in the mandible and on four implants in the maxilla have been shown to offer a significant improvement in function and retention (Fig 3.13a, b). Various forms of retention methods can be considered. However, it is important to solve the specific problems that the patient is experiencing. In this example, a removable dental prosthesis might remain uncomfortable in function, despite being implant-retained, if the patient has a very sensitive alveolar mucosa and a superficial mental nerve. In such cases, a fixed implant-supported prosthesis might be indicated that eliminates rubbing and pressure on the mucosa (Fig 3.13c–e).

Likewise, a patient with a gag reflex might continue to struggle with a removable prosthesis; hence, a fixed prosthesis might be better. Or, as illustrated in the example here, the palatal coverage of the prosthesis can be significantly reduced whilst enhancing retention (Fig 3.13f). This particular patient suffered from a severe gag reflex. A removable prosthesis with a labial flange was deemed appropriate to achieve the adequate lip support. A removable implant-supported and retained prosthesis was provided, and, simultaneously, the gag reflex was addressed by minimizing the palatal coverage.

Often, the patient wishes to avoid a removable dental prosthesis and prefers fixed tooth reconstructions. If, after thorough assessment, the alveolar bone height and width allow ideal implant positioning, then a fixed prosthesis can be provided. In this case, six implants were placed in the maxilla to support a full-arch fixed dental prosthesis (Fig 3.13g, h). Careful questioning is required to tease out the denture-related complaints of the patient and to ensure the treatment addresses them adequately and successfully.

There are certain clinical scenarios where it is not immediately obvious what the best combination of implants should be. These can be broadly categorized as:

- Replacing two adjacent teeth
- Replacing three adjacent teeth
- Replacing four or more adjacent teeth

### 3.14.1 Replacing Two Adjacent Teeth

The options in this case are to place two implants or a single implant. The decision will ultimately be made on how much space is available between the natural teeth mesial and distal to the edentulous space. Careful measurements need to be taken to ensure at least 1.5 mm of space is available between the implants and the natural teeth and at least 3 mm of space between implants. If there is insufficient space for two implants, a two-unit cantilever bridge using a single implant is recommended. This arrangement is particularly pertinent when replacing a central and a lateral incisor. More often, there is insufficient space to accommodate two implants in such a clinical scenario, and insufficient interimplant space will inevitably result in lack of papilla and consequently an aesthetic failure.

### 3.14.2 Replacing Three Adjacent Teeth

In this scenario, three implants are not indicated. Two implants supporting a fixed bridge is often adequate in this situation. The difficulty lies in deciding whether to place the implants adjacent to each other or mesially and distally in the space. Assessment of the alveolus in terms of volume of hard and soft tissues will inform the decision on where to place the implants. It is important to plan for this eventuality prior to commencing any surgery.

### 3.14.3 Replacing Four or More Adjacent Teeth

In these cases, the decision on where to place the implants is often difficult. Since these spans are large, spacing in between implants is unlikely to be an issue. Which sites to use for implant placement will be largely determined by the soft- and hard-tissue anatomy of the alveolus. Three-dimensional imaging cone beam CT scan can be extremely useful when planning long spans and should be considered in cases where multiple teeth are to be replaced

Treatment planning for implants requires a different set of diagnostic skills than planning for other types of dental treatment. It can seem complicated at first but with practice and experience will become second nature and will save time and frustration if carried out thoroughly. In summary, thorough planning is the key to successful outcomes in the aesthetic zone.

## References


1. Bain CA, Weng D, Meltzer A, Kohles SS, Stach RM. A meta-analysis evaluating the risk for implant failure in patients who smoke. Compend Contin Educ Dent. 2002;23(8):695–9. 704 passim; quiz 708.
2. Strietzel FP, Reichart PA, Kale A, Kulkarni M, Wegner B, Kuchler I. Smoking interferes with the prognosis of dental implant treatment: a systematic review and meta-analysis. J Clin Periodontol. 2007;34(6):523–44.
3. Heitz-Mayfield LJA, Huynh-Ba G. History of treated periodontitis and smoking as risks for implant therapy. Int J Oral Maxillofac Implants. 2009;24(Suppl):39–68.
4. Proceedings of the Third ITI (International Team for Implantology) Consensus Conference. Gstaad, Switzerland, August 2003. Int J Oral Maxillofac Implants. 2004;19(Suppl):7–154.
5. Ong CTT, Ivanovski S, Needleman IG, Retzepi M, Moles DR, Tonetti MS, et al. Systematic review of implant outcomes in treated periodontitis subjects. J Clin Periodontol. 2008;35(5):438–62.
6. Olsson M, Lindhe J, Marinello CP. On the relationship between crown form and clinical features of the gingiva in adolescents. J Clin Periodontol. 1993;20(8):570–7.
7. Evans CDJ, Chen ST. Esthetic outcomes of immediate implant placements. Clin Oral Implants Res. 2008;19(1):73–80.
8. Romeo E, Lops D, Rossi A, Storelli S, Rozza R, Chiapasco M. Surgical and prosthetic management of interproximal region with single-implant restorations: 1-year prospective study. J Periodontol. 2008;79(6):1048–55.
9. De Rouck T, Eghbali R, Collys K, De Bruyn H, Cosyn J. The gingival biotype revisited: transparency of the periodontal probe through the gingival margin as a method to discriminate thin from thick gingiva. J Clin Periodontol. 2009;36(5):428–33.
10. Lobbezoo F, Van Der Zaag J, Naeije M. Bruxism: its multiple causes and its effects on dental implants – an updated review. J Oral Rehabil. 2006;33(4):293–300.
11. Pjetursson BE, Tan K, Lang NP, Bragger U, Egger M, Zwahlen M. A systematic review of the survival and complication rates of fixed partial dentures (FPDs) after an observation period of at least 5 years. Clin Oral Implants Res. 2004;15(6):667–76.
12. Taylor TD, Wiens J, Carr A. Evidence-based considerations for removable prosthodontic and dental implant occlusion: a literature review. J Prosthet Dent. 2005;94(6):555–60.
13. Feine JS, Carlsson GE, Awad MA, Chehade A, Duncan WJ, Gizani S, et al. The McGill Consensus Statement on Overdentures. McGill University; 2002.
14. Thomason JM, Feine J, Exley C, Moynihan P, Müller F, et al. Mandibular Two Implant-Supported Overdentures as the First Choice Standard of Care for Edentulous Patients — The York Consensus Statement. Br Dent J. 2009;207:185–6.
15. Wu Y-J, Tu Y-K, Huang S-M, Chan C-P. The influence of the distance from the contact point to the crest of bone on the presence of the interproximal dental papilla. Chang Gung Med J. 2003;26(11):822–8.

16. Tarnow D, Elian N, Fletcher P, Froum S, Magner A, Cho S-C, et al. Vertical distance from the crest of bone to the height of the interproximal papilla between adjacent implants. J Periodontol. 2003;74(12):1785–8.
17. Tarnow DP, Cho SC, Wallace SS. The effect of inter-implant distance on the height of inter-implant bone crest. J Periodontol. 2000;71(4):546–9.
18. Esposito MAB, Koukoulopoulou A, Coulthard P, Worthington HV. Interventions for replacing missing teeth: dental implants in fresh extraction sockets (immediate, immediate-delayed and delayed implants). Cochrane Database Syst Rev. 2006;4:CD005968.
19. Botticelli D, Berglundh T, Lindhe J. Hard-tissue alterations following immediate implant placement in extraction sites. J Clin Periodontol. 2004;31(10):820–8.
20. Guerrero ME, Jacobs R, Loubele M, Schutyser F, Suetens P, van Steenberghe D. State-of-the-art on cone beam CT imaging for preoperative planning of implant placement. Clin Oral Investig. 2006;10(1):1–7.

## Further Reading

Levin L, Hertzberg R, Har-Nes S, Schwartz-Arad D. Long-term marginal bone loss around single dental implants affected by current and past smoking habits. Implant Dent. 2008;17(4):422–9.

Kao RT, Fagan MC, Conte GJ. Thick vs. thin gingival biotypes: a key determinant in treatment planning for dental implants. J Calif Dent Assoc. 2008;36(3):193–8.

Huynh-Ba G, Pjetursson BE, Sanz M, Cecchinato D, Ferrus J, Lindhe J, et al. Analysis of the socket bone wall dimensions in the upper maxilla in relation to immediate implant placement. Clin Oral Implants Res. 2010;21(1):37–42.

Esposito M, Grusovin MG, Coulthard P, Worthington HV. The efficacy of various bone augmentation procedures for dental implants: a Cochrane systematic review of randomized controlled clinical trials. Int J Oral Maxillofac Implants. 2006;21(5):696–710.

Belser UC, Grutter L, Vailati F, Bornstein MM, Weber H-P, Buser D. Outcome evaluation of early placed maxillary anterior single-tooth implants using objective esthetic criteria: a cross-sectional, retrospective study in 45 patients with a 2- to 4-year follow-up using pink and white esthetic scores. J Periodontol. 2009;80(1):140–51.

# Implant Surgery

# 4

Julian Yates

## 4.1 Introduction to Implant Surgery

The placement of dental implants involves a surgical procedure that facilitates the direct structural and functional connection between the jawbone (occasionally extra-oral bone) and the implant surface. The subsequent prostheses supported by the implant may include restorations such as crowns, bridges, over-dentures, orthodontic anchorage devices or facial prostheses. The biological process that occurs is referred to as osseointegration, whereby the surface of a load-bearing implant forms a direct and intimate interface with the bone. Healing time is required after the procedure, and, therefore, the clinicians involved in the surgery must follow strict patient care principles during and after the surgery to guarantee an optimal recovery. During surgery, the nature and position of the implant is determined by the quantity and quality of the bone present, along with the desired implant size (length and width), the position of adjacent teeth (if present) and the requirements of the planned prosthesis. The provision of dental implants should be driven by a prosthetic requirement and therefore delivered with utmost precision in order to obtain an optimal dental or restorative outcome for the patient. Generally, dental implants are used to replace one or more missing teeth lost by dental decay, trauma, periodontal disease, surgical excision or in cases where teeth are congenitally missing and where conventional avenues of treatment have either been exhausted, are not possible or cannot be provided with any degree of predictability. Given the pattern of tooth loss, it is essential that both the restorative and surgical requirements of the patient are considered together prior to treatment.

J. Yates (✉)
Oral Surgery, Division of Dentistry, School of Medical Sciences, University of Manchester, Manchester, UK
e-mail: julian.yates@manchester.ac.uk



C. Barclay (ed.), *Oral Implantology: Assessment to Maintenance*, BDJ Clinician's Guides, https://doi.org/10.1007/978-3-031-55241-0_4

Over the last few decades, dental implantology has gained increasing popularity and is currently experiencing an increase in growth due to the demands and expectations of patients, and also the desire to continually improve patients' quality of life.

## 4.2 Scope of Practice and Competency

The scope of practice for implant surgeons is broad and encompasses many aspects of surgical and restorative care, both in general terms, and directly relating to implantology. Whilst there are transferable skills, there are also specific skills relating to implantology that need to be acquired. As such, clinicians must attain training and competencies that translate to their scope of practice. Dental implantology involves patient assessment, diagnosis and treatment planning for the provision of an implant, or other dental restorative procedures relating to the provision of dental implants. Therefore, given the potential complexities of this modality of treatment, clinicians must also be able to evaluate patients critically, noting the existence of comorbidities, and have the ability to advise on how and when implant treatment can be best undertaken. In such scenarios, or during the patient evaluation, an appreciation of clinical, medical or social conditions that a patient may present with is critical, as some may negatively affect the provision of dental implants, both in the short and long term.

The provision of dental implants has revolutionized dental training and competency-based education. Apart from basic education and training, dental surgeons are now involved in training to boost competence and skills in order to undertake dental implant surgery [1]. The training of an implant dentist is offered in hospitals, clinics/practices, Royal Colleges and universities. In the United Kingdom, the General Dental Council regulations require that dental graduates are able to perform routine exodontia, simple minor oral surgery procedures and an array of restorative treatments. Dental implantology, however, requires a level of post-graduate training in order to achieve the level of competency necessary to safely provide such treatment. That is not to say a single level of competence is required, as the emphasis is placed on the clinician to determine the level of complexity they wish to progress to. The standards developed by the FGDP "Training standards in implant dentistry" (2016) provide guidance on the level of competency required for implant dentistry to assure patient safety. Competence is evaluated through the successful management of patients before, during and after implant provision (Seward 2018), through patient satisfaction and continuous medical education.

## 4.3 Patient Selection, Management of the Medically Compromised Patient and Treatment Planning

Before a clinician undertakes implant treatment, it is essential they develop competence in procedures including clinical assessment, treatment planning, implant placement and restoration. The knowledge and skills relevant to treatment planning are acquired during training and through experience, and clinicians must be ready to make appropriate decisions and evaluate whether implant treatment is indicated or contraindicated in specific circumstances. It must be remembered that implant treatment is not appropriate for all patients. The first step in the treatment planning process is to assess if the patient is suitable or able to undergo treatment through a risk–benefit analysis and identify any underlying conditions (local or systemic) that may negatively influence the outcomes of the treatment proposed. Examples of these can be seen in Table 4.1.

The clinician must then determine the complexity of the case and communicate this with the patient, informing them of the treatment proposed, any possible alternatives, and the risks and benefits involved with the treatment suggested in order to obtain valid consent.

As well as conditions listed in Table 4.1, other contraindications may include patients with acute infectious conditions, incomplete tooth eruption, allergies or reactions to certain materials, poor oral hygiene or an ability to maintain optimal oral hygiene. Clinicians must thoroughly assess patients and note any contraindications in order to avoid exposing patients to excessive risks. Within the United Kingdom, the Association of Dental Implantology (ADI) has published advice on cases where special consideration should be given prior to providing dental implants [2]. These considerations include

- Radiation to the jaws
- Untreated intra-oral dental disease, pathology or malignancy
- Untreated periodontal disease
- Uncontrolled drug or alcohol use (abuse)
- Uncontrolled psychiatric disorders
- Significant medical events, including recent myocardial infarction (MI), cerebrovascular accident (CVA), valvular prostheses surgery, or other events that may negatively influence healing of the patients and their ability to withstand or recover from surgery
- IV bisphosphonate therapy
- Immunosuppression including post-organ transplantation or presence or treatment of other systemic disease
- Inability to maintain high levels of plaque control (reduced manual dexterity and failure to engage with cleaning)

**Table 4.1** Medical conditions that may affect the provision and successful outcome of implant treatment

| Medical condition | Implications for treatment delivery | Recommendation |
|---|---|---|
| Cardiovascular<br>Uncontrolled hypertension<br>Angina<br>Recent MI<br>Cardiac defects/valve replacement/ previous endocarditis/ | Risk of bleeding<br>Failure to clot or difficulty in clotting<br>Excessive bruising<br>Susceptibility to adrenaline-containing LA or anxiety-induced chest pain<br>Risk of MI<br>Repeat MI<br>Increased risk with adrenaline-containing LA<br>Development of infective endocarditis | >180/100—referral to medical practitioner for urgent assessment—this is their priority in terms of healthcare<br>>160/100—consider local measures to reduce bleeding<br>Up to 160/100—treat as normal<br>Have GNT spray and oxygen available<br>If patient is successfully treated (i.e. stents, CABG) or has recovered—treat as normal<br>Consider delay in elective treatment with LA by up to 3 months<br>Consider delay in elective treatment by GA by up to 6 months<br>Be aware of concurrent anti-coagulant therapy post-MI and manage appropriately<br>Antibiotic cover for prevention of endocarditis not recommended<br>Consider whether antibiotic prophylaxis is required for the surgical procedure—if so, use appropriate anti-microbial therapy |
| Respiratory –<br>Asthma<br>COPD<br>URTI | Difficulty in tolerating surgery—positioning<br>Anxiety may worsen conditions<br>Provision of analgesics may impact respiratory conditions. i.e. aspirin and NSAIDs may exacerbate asthma<br>Steroids used for respiratory conditions may limit use of NSAIDs and Aspirin and increase risk of gastric ulceration<br>Certain medications used to treat severe asthma may affect liver and cardiac function | Consider suitability for surgery—posture/positioning, length, complexity of procedure<br>Patients should bring inhalers in case of acute episodes of asthma or to optimize COPD<br>IVS may help with anxiety-induced asthma<br>IVS and GA may not be suitable for patients with COPD<br>If on long-term steroids for respiratory condition, consider appropriate post-operative analgesics, i.e. paracetamol or compound analgesics<br>Steroid cover may be required for patients on high-dose steroids to avoid hypotensive crisis<br>Be aware of drug interactions—leukotriene receptor antagonists may impair liver function (increase the risk of bleeding) whilst theophylline may exaggerate effect of adrenaline in LA (induce cardiac arrythmias) |

| | | |
|---|---|---|
| Haematological disorders –<br>Haemophilia A, B, von Willebrand's<br>Thrombocytopenia<br>Anti-coagulant therapy (warfarin, aspirin, clopidogrel, or other novel oral anti-coagulants) | Significant risk of bleeding<br>Significant risk of bleeding<br>Significant risk of bleeding | Implant surgery is considered a procedure that carries a higher risk of bleeding<br>Patient will be known by local haematology service if diagnosed. May require infusions of appropriate blood clotting factors or DDAVP.<br>Patients with a history of thrombocytopenia will require input from haematology services<br>• If platelet levels are <50 × $10^{-9}$/L, patient will require platelet infusion<br>• If platelet levels are >50 × $10^{-9}$/L, consider local measures to reduce post-operative bleeding<br>• Consider tranexamic acid or DDAVP<br>• Avoid analgesics such as aspirin and NSAIDs<br>Follow SDCEP guidance<br>Warfarin –<br>Pre-operative INR (within 24 h if unstable or 72 h if stable)<br>INR >4—delay treatment<br>INR <4—proceed as normal but monitor<br>Consider limiting treatment, i.e. staged approach<br>Consider providing local measures to reduce risk of bleeding<br>Do not alter INR levels—refer to treating doctor to adjust to appropriate levels<br>Anti-platelet drugs (single/dual therapy) –<br>Consider limiting treatment i.e. staged approach<br>Consider providing local measures to reduce risk of bleeding<br>Expect delay in clotting<br>Novel oral anti-coagulant – Advise patient to miss (apixaban, dabigatran)/delay (rivaroxaban) their morning dose on the day of their surgical procedure<br>Consider limiting treatment, i.e. staged approach<br>Consider providing local measures to reduce risk of bleeding<br>Advice when to restart medication<br>Injectable anti-coagulant –<br>Seek specialist advice |

(continued)

**Table 4.1** (continued)

| Medical condition | Implications for treatment delivery | Recommendation |
|---|---|---|
| Liver disease –<br>Non-alcoholic fatty liver disease<br>Alcohol-related liver disease<br>Viral liver disease/hepatitis—Hep A, B, C<br>Haemochromatosis<br>Primary biliary cirrhosis | Risk of bleeding—abnormal clotting factors<br>Altered drug metabolism<br>Cross-infection risk—Hep A, B, C, D, E | Request FBC, LFT and clotting profile to assess liver function<br>Consider limiting treatment, i.e. staged approach<br>Consider providing local measures to reduce risk of bleeding<br>Check dosages of prescribed medications<br>Cross-infection |
| Kidney disease –<br>Chronic kidney conditions | Risk of bleeding—abnormal platelet numbers/thrombocytopenia<br>Altered drug metabolism<br>Infection—susceptible to infection at end-stage kidney disease or may be on immune-suppressants post-transplant | Request FBC and U&E's in severe cases to assess kidney function<br>Check dosages of prescribed medications<br>Consider whether antibiotic prophylaxis is required for the surgical procedure—if so, use appropriate anti-microbial therapy |
| Diabetes –<br>Poorly controlled Type I or II diabetes | Care when planning for elective surgery, i.e. timing, appropriate glycaemic control, hypoglycaemic episode<br>Increased risk of infection and poor healing due to effect on white blood cells, fibroblasts and other cells involved in the healing process.<br>General systemic upset—poorly controlled | Assess glycaemic control prior to elective surgery –<br>Acute control –<br>Target blood sugar levels –<br>Pre-meal—4– 7 mmol/L for patients with type I and type II diabetes<br>After meals—under 9 mmol/L for people with type 1 diabetes and under 8.5 mmol/L for people with type 2 diabetes<br>Chronic control—HbA1c<br>Normal—Below 42 mmol/mol<br>Prediabetes—42 to 47 mmol/mol<br>Diabetes—48 mmol/mol<br>Elective surgery should be avoided in patients with HbA1c levels over 55 mmol/mol due to increased risk of infection and non-healing |
| Epilepsy | Poorly controlled epilepsy or anxiety may increase risk of seizure | Check control of epilepsy<br>If poorly controlled, request treating physician to optimize control<br>If poorly controlled or with specific triggers relating to stress/anxiety. consider treatment with IVS or GA in a controlled environment |

| | | |
|---|---|---|
| Uncontrolled alcohol/drug abuse | Risk of bleeding—abnormal clotting factors<br>Altered drug metabolism<br>Cross-infection risk—Hep A, B, C, D, E<br>Difficulty providing adequate analgesia | Request FBC, LFT and clotting profile to assess liver function<br>Consider limiting treatment i.e. staged approach<br>Consider providing local measures to reduce risk of bleeding<br>Check dosages of prescribed medications<br>Cross-infection<br>Seek advice on peri-operative analgesia—if possible, avoid opiates due to alcohol dependence, self-prescribing (benzodiazepines or opiates) or taking regular replacement therapy for withdrawals |
| HIV | Systemic –<br>Viral load and CD4 count may influence suitability for surgery<br>Thrombocytopenia<br>Cross-infection risk<br>Condition of soft tissues—presence of HIV-associated oral mucosal conditions may preclude patient form surgery, candidiasis, oral hairy leukoplakia, recurrent herpes simplex infections, recurrent apthae/ulcers, periodontal disease and xerostomia. | Viral load low (<50 RNA copies/ml blood)—low infection risk—elective implant treatment possible<br>CD4 count—>200 cells/μL blood—adequate immune system—elective implant treatment possible<br>See haematological disorders<br>Cross-infection<br>Avoid elective treatment if soft tissues are compromised |
| Chemotherapy | Ability to withstand surgery –<br>Risk of bleeding due to thrombocytopenia<br>Risk of infection due to neutropenia<br>General systemic upset | Cyclical events associated with chemotherapy may mean surgery is not appropriate during and immediately after chemotherapy rounds. However, windows of opportunity may be available between cycles—will require haematological investigations to determine suitability<br>See haematological disorders<br>Consider anti-microbial cover peri-operatively<br>Not suitable for elective surgery—await outcome of chemotherapy |

(continued)

**Table 4.1** (continued)

| Medical condition | Implications for treatment delivery | Recommendation |
| --- | --- | --- |
| Radiotherapy | Risk of osteoradionecrosis (ORN) following surgery—has the radiotherapy involved the site to be treated or possibly elsewhere<br>Patient receiving radiotherapy for curative or palliative intent.<br>Risk of ORN following surgery is greater in patients who have<br>• received a total dose of >60Gy<br>• radiation involving the primary site<br>Radiotherapy affects implant success both pre- and post-radiotherapy<br>• implants placed in areas of dose <45 Gy appear to have a more favourable outcome than those >45 Gy<br>• short- and long-term survival may be affected by effects of radiotherapy on the surrounding tissues<br>General systemic upset<br>Risk of infection | Assess radiotherapy field—request planning images<br>Determine the dose given at the site of proposed treatment<br>Is treatment appropriate<br>Detail increase risks for ORN and implant failure<br>Referral to specialist centre for planning and treatment<br>Not suitable for elective surgery—await outcome of radiotherapy<br>Consider anti-microbial cover peri-operatively |

| Bisphosphonates and other anti-angiogenic medications, e.g. denosumab | Risk of MRONJ—related to dose, duration and method of administration<br>Low risk—<3 years of oral therapy with no other medical issues relating to immunosuppression or steroid use.<br>Moderate risk—>3 years of oral therapy with other medical issues relating to immunosuppression or steroid use or IV MRONJ therapy<br>High risk—high-dose IV therapy with other medical issues relating to immunosuppression or steroid use | Low risk—detail additional risks and treat as normal<br>Moderate/high risk—not suitable for elective implant treatment<br>If undergoing implant therapy, consider peri-operative mouthwash and anti-microbials |
|---|---|---|
| Immunosuppression<br>Common mediations—methotrexate, azathioprine, infliximab, leflunomide, high dose steroids | Identify reason for reduced immunity—medication-related, chemotherapy, radiotherapy, viral, endocrine<br>Ability to withstand surgery<br>Risk of bleeding due to thrombocytopenia<br>Risk of infection due to neutropenia<br>General systemic upset | May consider drug "holiday" to reduce risks but need to balance issues with worsening of condition/symptoms<br>Evidence stronger for some medications than others<br>Consider staged approach or modified treatment plan to reduce surgical insult<br>See haematological disorders<br>Consider peri-operative anti-microbials<br>Timing of elective surgery—may need to delay |
| Uncontrolled psychiatric conditions | Issues relating to –<br>Understanding processes/procedures<br>Expectations<br>Consent<br>Disproportionate responses to surgical or prosthetic issues | Consent process—more detailed explanation and alternative ways of presenting information<br>Address and change expectations—if possible<br>Elective implant treatment may not be appropriate |

Once a clinical assessment has been completed, the patient should then have the appropriate images and pre-treatment records taken for planning and guiding an appropriate treatment plan. With a plan in place and valid consent obtained, the clinician can plan and prepare for the surgical stage, which will involve the acquisition of the various implants and components, as well as the surgical materials and necessary equipment.

## 4.4 Basic Surgical Principles and Pre-Operative Preparation

Dental implantology is guided by basic surgical principles applied to the process of osseointegration combined with the aim of achieving optimal functional and aesthetic outcomes. The principles include that the clinician must possess appropriate skills and knowledge in surgery, prosthodontics and the biomechanical principles relating to dentistry. The dental team must also follow appropriate protocols for the management of patients pre-, during and post-dental implant surgery to help promote safe and effective patient care, improved recovery and achieve optimal clinical outcomes. The provision of dental implantology is not restricted to any one aspect of patient care, and the dental team should follow an integrated and holistic approach to managing the patient throughout their treatment pathway.

## 4.5 Informed and Valid Consent

Prior to any surgery, it is essential that valid consent has been obtained in order to demonstrate that the patient has been informed not only of the procedure itself but also of any alternative treatments available, and the risks and benefits of the treatment proposed and any potential complications that may arise from providing the treatment. Consent is part of the legal and ethical requirements for a patient preparing to undergo surgery or a complex medical procedure and is an essential element of the GDC's Standards for the dental team. Ideally, written consent signed by the patient and clinician responsible for the treatment should be obtained, as this would provide details of the discussions that took place. Informed consent can only be obtained after patient discussions and education, and the person obtaining the consent for the proposed implant surgery should be familiar with the procedure and know the potential hazards. The patient should have adequate time to consider the proposed treatment, have sufficient information to make an informed choice and not been influenced or coerced in such a way that they feel pressured into undergoing treatment. The patient must, therefore, reflect and make any decision independently. If the patient is not conversant with the language of the consent form, a translator for that language should be used so that the patient understands what the whole process will involve.

## 4.6 Considerations Following Tooth Loss

Following tooth loss, alveolar bone undergoes remodelling and resorption, which can lead to a reduction in the quantity and quality of hard tissue available for implant placement. The process of resorption can lead to reduced volumes of hard and soft tissues both horizontally and vertically, which may compromise the ideal positioning of any dental implant.

Residual bone quantity will determine the length and diameter of the implant that can be placed for the provision of a prosthesis, and if insufficient, augmentation or grafting may have to be undertaken. Lekholm and Zarb [3] provided one of the earliest classifications of bone remodelling following tooth loss, and further modifications have also demonstrated changes in the quality of the bone that exists. Figure 4.1 illustrates the horizontal and vertical changes that occur during resorption as well as the different proportions of the cortical and cancellous bone that are present in different individuals. Whilst a reduction in bone volume may negatively influence the position of any intended dental implant, the quality will influence the surgical protocol used when undertaking surgery to place an implant.

Bone quality may be characterized by the amounts of cortical and cancellous bone present at the surgical site. Differences in the quality of bone present will lead

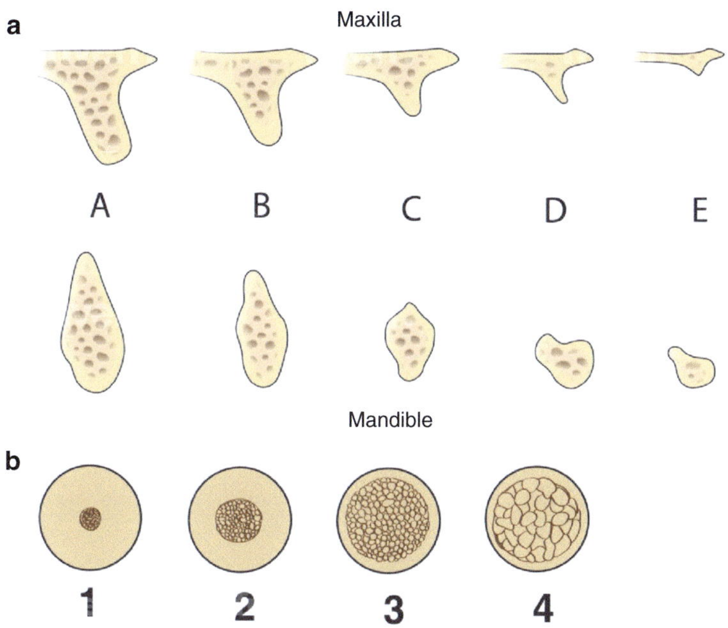


**Fig. 4.1** Diagrammatic illustration representing: (**a**) the patterns of resorption in the maxilla and mandible following tooth loss—from minimal to extreme; (**b**) distribution and proportions of cortical (outer layer) and cancellous (inner layer) present in bone. The overall classification can be determined as any combination of the two characteristics highlighted. (Modified form [3])

to changes in drill selection, osteotomy preparation and implant insertion and survival. The presence of minimal cortical bone and a relatively large proportion of cancellous bone may mean that osteotomy preparation has to be reduced relative to the dimensions of the implant so that adequate primary stability can be obtained. Conversely, in cases where cortical bone is abundant, the osteotomy site may have to be over-prepared relative to the implant dimension, and even supplemented with bone-tapping techniques in order to prevent damage to either the implant or the surrounding bone during insertion.

Where bone volume has reduced beyond the ideal, the quantity, quality and proportion of augmented or grafted bone will determine the number and position of implants placed, and for any given prosthetic scenario, there is no pre-determined number of implants required. Whilst the number of implants required for single teeth and small spanning bridges may be relatively simple to determine, patients requiring full-arch fixed or removable prostheses may require fewer fixtures where there is adequate quantity and optimal quality of hard tissues, when compared to patients who have reduced volumes and sub-optimal quality of bone. There is strong debate around the "ideal" numbers of implants required for full-arch restorations; however, for many clinicians, this is based not only on the availability of hard and soft issues, but also on their preferred treatment protocol.

## 4.7 Implant Surgery

Prior to any implant surgery, it is imperative that all the materials and equipment are available to undertake the proposed treatment and that adequate time is given to complete the surgery. This is especially the case when first embarking upon implant surgery or undertaking complex cases. To provide safe and effective treatment, the details given in Table 4.2 should be considered.

**Table 4.2** Peri-operative considerations for the provision of safe and effective implant treatment

| | |
|---|---|
| Time | Is there adequate time for the procedure<br>Does the time allow for:<br>• detailing the proposed treatment<br>• confirmation of consent<br>• provision of pre-operative medications, i.e. antibiotics, mouthwash<br>• undertaking the treatment/surgery<br>• provision of temporary prosthesis<br>• provision of immediate restorations<br>• discussing post-operative care<br>• cleaning down the surgery<br>• arranging for review appointments |
| Surgical/restorative aids | Imaging—2D or 3D<br>Study models<br>Surgical guides/stents<br>Diagnostic wax-up<br>Temporary prostheses |
| Surgical and implant kits | Appropriate sterile surgical equipment Appropriate/correct implant kit<br>Correct-sized dental implants<br>Sutures<br>Augmentation material |
| Aseptic environment | Surgical gowns<br>Surgical drapes<br>Surgery preparation |
| Pre-operative medications | Antibiotics and/or mouth rinse |
| Local anaesthetic | Short-acting LA—is the proposed treatment short and being undertaken by an experienced operator<br>Long-acting LA—is the procedure long or being undertaken by an inexperienced operator<br>Repeat LA |
| IVS—if treatment will be undertaken with sedation | Additional consent<br>Time for preparation, i.e. cannulation, baseline observations<br>Time for recovery<br>Post-operative instruction, i.e. escort<br>Mobilization of the patient |
| Post-operative care | Post-operative advice to patient<br>Arrangements for review |
| Documentation | Completion of notes—these may be more complex than normal<br>Filing/scanning of additional documentation<br>Detailing and recording components and materials used<br>Completion of laboratory prescription<br>Ordering new components/materials |

## 4.8 Implant Planning and Surgical Preparation

*Prosthetically driven surgery*: From the outset, it must be remembered that the provision of dental implants is driven by the requirements of the planned prosthesis and not purely by the availability of soft and hard tissues alone, and therefore, it is a restoratively or prosthetically driven concept. Utilizing backward planning or the "crown down" concept, with the proposed prosthesis in mind, an appropriate number of implants and their ideal positions can be determined in order to obtain an optimal outcome. Depending on the availability of bone, additional regenerative techniques, including guided bone regeneration (GBR) or formal block bone grafting, may be required in order to achieve this objective. On some occasions, this can be undertaken simultaneously with implant placement; however, on other occasions, augmentation/grafting may need to be completed prior to implant placement in order to prepare the surgical site for optimal implant positioning.

In order to plan for optimal implant placement, it is recommended that in all but the simplest of cases, a surgical stent/guide should be used to aid osteotomy preparation. The production of a surgical stent/guide can be undertaken using both traditional analogue techniques and more recent digital methods. In recent years, with the increasing use of digital scanning techniques and cone beam CT technology, there has been a move towards digital pathways for prosthesis design, implant planning and surgical placement.

*Surgical principles:* Following initial preparation of the patient, implant surgery involves five principle steps—provision of anaesthesia, soft-tissue incision and reflection, low-speed drilling and osteotomy preparation, implant placement and soft-tissue approximation and closure. It is important when undertaking soft-tissue surgery that incisions are made with respect to important anatomical structures and standard flap design, in order to provide adequate exposure of the surgical site and to allow manipulation of the gingiva to provide a band of keratinized mucosa on both the buccal and lingual/palatal aspects of the implant and transmucosal element of the final implant-retained prosthesis.

Osteotomy preparation is usually undertaken with drilling speeds between 500 and 1500 rpm with copious irrigation using standard saline solution, although this is dependent on the drilling protocol used. Care should be taken not to exceed these drilling speeds, as handling of the drills during osteotomy preparation can become difficult, and overheating and subsequent necrosis of the bone can occur. Ideally, drilling is undertaken using a stent or a surgical guide to place the pilot hole in the appropriate position, although experience may dictate if this is required for simple or routine cases. Drilling is undertaken to establish the length required for the planned implant, and the initial (pilot) hole is then expanded using increasingly wider drills to the appropriate size for the implant system used. The exact osteotomy size will be determined by the requirements of the specific implant system used and the quantity and quality of the bone available. Placement of the implant is usually undertaken by slowly screwing the implant into the osteotomy at speeds between 25 and 50 rpm, in a self-tapping manner. In the majority of the cases, drilling of the bone produces an osteotomy site that is marginally smaller than the implant, with the aim of establishing adequate primary stability to encourage successful osseointegration. However, as detailed previously, in some cases, the size of the final osteotomy may need to be reduced or increased, relative to the size of the planned implant, depending on the quality of the hard tissues. Finally, tissue closure is undertaken to adapt the gingiva either over or around the implant site, thereby establishing a covering of healthy keratinized mucosa.

*Timing of implant surgery:* The timing of implant placement can vary depending on the treatment protocol used and can be defined as either immediate, early or late implant placement. Late implant placement may occur in instances where tooth loss happened many months or years prior to the patient considering implant treatment. Early placement can be where a delay in treatment has been electively chosen due to the presence of long-term infection, pathology or unstable and disrupted tissues following tooth removal, whilst immediate implant placement involves preparation of the osteotomy and placement of the implant at the time of tooth extraction. Whilst the latter may be possible in some instances, where the anatomy is favourable for implants to be placed within fresh extraction sockets (incisor, canine and pre-molar teeth); on some occasions, it is not possible due to the unfavourable nature of the surgical site (molar teeth).

Both methods have their advantages and disadvantages. The delayed approach will allow implant placement into healed and mature hard and soft tissues and, therefore, arguably, provide a more predictable outcome. However, the disadvantages are that there will be an inevitable delay in treatment and a risk of hard and soft tissue resorption following tooth loss, which may influence the position on any future implants, and necessitate additional augmentation and grafting. The advantages of immediate implant placement are that the patient is exposed to fewer surgical episodes, and the overall treatment time is reduced. There is also evidence to suggest that success rates are comparable to those with a delayed approach, and that it may also help to preserve soft and hard tissue morphology following tooth extraction. Conversely, there are studies that demonstrate immediate placement can be associated with a higher frequency of bony defects presenting as abutment or implant exposure, although these can be largely prevented with appropriate augmentation at the time of placement.

The technique of immediate and delayed implant placement can also be divided into one-stage and two-stage placements. One-stage (or single-stage) placement is where the implant is placed along with a transmucosal abutment, which is slightly above the soft tissues and does not require further surgery to expose it. Two-stage placement is where the implant is placed with a sub-mucosal cover screw. This technique will require further surgery in order to expose the implant and provide either a transmucosal healing abutment or temporary or definitive prosthesis. The two-stage technique may be used in cases where the soft and hard tissues are compromised, additional augmentation or grafting techniques are needed, or where the predictability of the outcome needs to be broadened.

*Implant size, position and angulation:* Prosthetic design and hard tissue quantity and quality will largely determine the length, diameter, position, angulation and drilling protocol employed for implant placement. Historically, the aim was to use all of the available bone, as well as the longest possible implant with bi-cortical anchorage, to provide the maximum level of primary and secondary stability. However, in recent years, there has been a move away from this thinking towards a more conservative approach. Most implant manufacturers provide a range of implant lengths and diameters, and an appropriately sized fixture should be used depending on the clinical scenario. However, the idea of placing the "largest implant possible" has been replaced with providing a suitably sized fixture with the aim of maintaining as much bone and soft tissue around the implant as reasonably possible in order to maintain tissue viability and improve its long-term stability.

When undertaking surgery to place dental implants, consideration must be given to both the horizontal and vertical positions of the fixture as well as its angulation in relation to the planned prosthesis and adjacent anatomical structures. Importantly, osteotomy preparation and implant placement is a three-dimensional concept that requires careful planning and execution in order to achieve treatment success and optimal long-term outcomes.

When considering the size of an implant, a minimum thickness of 1.5–2 mm of bone should be preserved around the implant in order to provide adequate hard-tissue stability, otherwise there is a risk that resorption can occur, leading to exposure of the trans-mucosal element of the restoration or the implant threads. A minimum distance of approximately 3 mm should also be maintained between implants in order to allow for adequate spacing between restorations and to provide a suitable environment that does not compromise the soft and hard tissues between the implants. Similar spacing should also be employed between natural teeth and implants to avoid damaging the adjacent roots and help maintain the inter-proximal bone between the fixture and the tooth, which in turn will help support the soft tissues, including the inter-dental papillae (Fig. 4.2).

In relation to the horizontal positioning of the osteotomy preparation and implant placement, care must be taken not to place the fixture too buccal or palatal. Ideally,

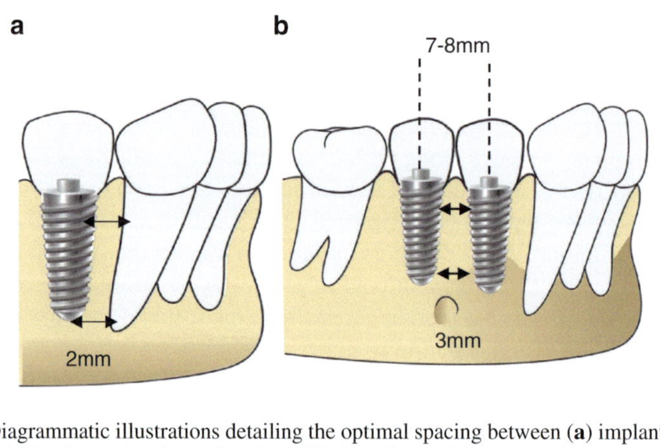


**Fig. 4.2** Diagrammatic illustrations detailing the optimal spacing between (**a**) implants and natural teeth and (**b**) adjacent implants. Spacing will allow for optimal prosthetic outcomes as well as preserving soft and hard tissues

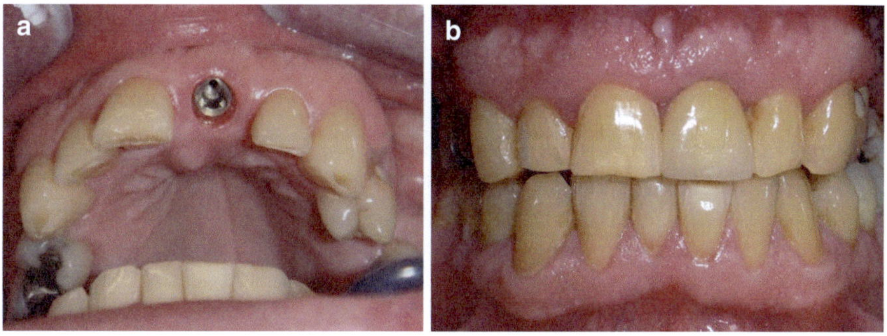


**Fig. 4.3** Clinical photographs detailing: (**a**) horizontal position of the implant within the "prosthetic envelope" of the adjacent teeth and to a vertical height that allows for an adequate emergence profile for the restoration (soft-tissue height approximately 4–5 mm; (**b**) restored implant showing correct position and appropriate soft-tissue emergence of the restoration to help support the adjacent soft tissue

the position should be within the "prosthetic envelope" of the planned prosthesis so that it position does not adversely affect the design, construction or emergence of the prosthesis (Fig. 4.3). With regards to vertical positioning of the dental implant, the optimal position for the head of the fixture is approximately 1–2 mm below the cemento-enamel junction of the adjacent tooth, as this will provide adequate height for an optimal emergence profile for the planned restoration in relation to the adjacent teeth. Where there is recession around adjacent teeth, either the position of the implant will have to be changed, and placed more apically, or additional procedures will have to be undertaken to address the soft- and hard-tissue deficiencies so that an optimal aesthetic outcome is achieved. Where adjacent teeth are not present, a height of 4–5 mm below the mucosal surface will suffice.

Fixture angulation is another important consideration when placing dental implants. Ideally, implants should be placed in an axial position in order to adequately accommodate the occlusal forced delivered through any planned prosthesis. However, in some clinical situations, it may be acceptable to tilt or angle dental implants in order that they do not encroach upon important anatomical structures or adjacent teeth. It has been reported that non-axial implants have comparable success rates to axially positioned implants, and indeed some treatment protocols require that implants are deliberately placed non-axially in order to do just that (i.e. all-on-4 concept).

Following tooth loss, pronounced hard-tissue resorption can occur, which can lead to a reduction in the width of the alveolus, primarily on the buccal aspect. This can occur in both the maxilla and mandible, but is more prominent towards the anterior region of the jaws. These concavities can be significant if tooth loss was as a result of trauma or surgery to deal with any dental or bony pathology in the region. In order to compensate for this hard-tissue loss, it may be possible to angle implants towards a more palatable position apically in order to engage the hard tissues and avoid dehiscence of the buccal bone plate, should a more axial position be attempted.

On many occasions, the compensation afforded by such a modified approach is limited, and where bone loss has occurred, augmentation or grafting may still be required.

Another consideration when determining the angulation of an implant during surgery is the requirement for either a cement- or screw-retained prosthesis. When planning for a screw-retained prosthesis, the screw access hole should be in alignment with the long axis of the implant and placed palatal/lingual to the incisal edge or cingulum, or within the occlusal surface of the restoration in order to achieve an optimal outcome in terms of axial loading and aesthetics. However, this may not be possible due to the presence of hard-tissue loss or significant buccal concavities, and therefore, a cement-retaining restoration may have to be considered. In cases where cement-retained restorations are planned, or necessary, the angulation of the fixture is less critical, as any move away from a true axial position may be corrected by the transmucosal abutment.

When planning the ideal position for any potential implant, specific consideration should be given to the requirements laid out by the implant manufacturer, as different systems employ different strategies to help maintain hard and soft tissues and enhance the emergence profile of any given prosthesis (i.e. platform switching, tissue-level implants); therefore, the horizontal and vertical positions of any fixture placed may vary according to the requirements of the system. Furthermore, the positional requirements for single-unit or small-span restorations will be different from those for larger prostheses, especially where atrophy of the hard and soft tissues is present. The former may require more accurate positioning of implants in order not to adversely affect the aesthetic outcome, whereas with full-arch restorations, where atrophy is present, there may be an element of flexibility when determining where fixtures should be placed.

## 4.9 Post-Operative Care: Once Surgery Is Complete

Following implant surgery, the patient can expect to be in some discomfort for several days. There is evidence to suggest clinicians routinely underestimate the discomfort patients can be in following surgery, and so attention should be given to how this can be managed best. The discomfort will usually last 3–5 days, but can be longer if additional procedures have been undertaken, including augmentation and grafting. The discomfort experienced can usually be managed with regular analgesics, and ideally, pain medication should be started when the effects of the local anaesthetic start to dissipate. Evidence suggests that for optimal pain relief, compound analgesia should be provided in the form of paracetamol and ibuprofen, at the recommended dose, if the patient can tolerate these medications.

It is also important that for the first 5–7 days after surgery, the patient maintains optimal oral hygiene. This can be undertaken by using regular anti-microbial mouthwash such as chlorhexidine, although warm salty mouthwash has also been shown to be beneficial post-surgery. Tooth brushing should be avoided for 24 h after surgery to prevent disturbance of the surgical site and allow the tissues to repair. As highlighted, swelling can be significant after implant surgery, and patients should be advised that this is a normal occurrence and not be unduly worried. However, if the swelling does not improve or becomes hard and hot to touch, then further investigations may be warranted and anti-microbial therapy may need to be started if there is evidence of infection.

In the vast majority of cases, resorbable sutures are used to approximate soft tissues following implant placement. However, there is an increasing trend for monofilament non-resorbable sutures to be used in order to prevent post-operative inflammation and infection. Whilst the former will "dissolve", the latter will have to be removed. In either case, some sutures can persist and be problematic for patients. In this situation, sutures can be removed after 5–7 days, as they will have performed their role by this time.

In relation to the provision of anti-microbials and implant treatment, there is significant debate as to whether they benefit the patient and enhance osseointegration and short-term outcomes following implant placement. There is some evidence to suggest that a single pre-operative dose of anti-microbials may reduce the risk of implant failure in normal conditions, with far less evidence available to support the use of anti-microbial therapy post-operatively. However, it is acknowledged that the threshold for provision is lowered when additional procedures are undertaken, including augmentation and grafting. There is no clear consensus as to which antimicrobial provides the most benefit for patients undergoing implant therapy, although routine prophylactic measures are usually adopted based on the knowledge we have in dealing with routine oral surgery and oro-facial infections.

## 4.10 Conclusion

Dental implantology is a rapidly growing field in dentistry; however, the delivery of such care requires a high level of competence, thorough training and experience in several aspects of dentistry. The swift growth has been influenced by several factors, including the availability of training and equipment required to undertake such procedures, the demand by patients and their ability to replace missing teeth in a way that conventional removable prostheses often cannot. The provision of such treatment entails meticulous pre-operative, operative and post-operative planning to ensure the procedure is effective, and optimal long-term clinical outcomes and patient satisfaction can be achieved.

## References


1. Piconi C, Sandri M. Key engineering materials. Trans Tech Publ. 2017.
2. ADI - Special considerations for imant treatment. 2019. https://www.adi.org.uk/_userfiles/pages/files/dental_implant_placement_guidelines_mar_23.pdf.
3. Lekholm U, Zarb GA. In: Branemark PI, Zarb GA, Albrektsson T, editors. Patient selection and preparation. Tissue integrated prostheses: osseointegration in clinical dentistry. Chicago: Quintessence Publishing Company; 1985. p. 199–209.

# 5 Managing Soft-Tissue/Bone Deficiency

Patrick Palacci

## 5.1 Introduction

Aesthetic considerations with regards to the soft and hard tissues around dental implants, particularly in the aesthetic zone, should receive as much attention as the placement and restoration of the implant itself. In today's society, patients have increasingly high expectations and aesthetic requirements. In order to achieve optimal aesthetic and biological results, optimisation of the soft and hard tissues around dental implants is often indicated.

Success of the dental implant treatment depends on four main factors:

- Management of hard tissue
- Management of soft tissue
- Quality of the prosthetic restoration
- Precision in implant positioning

Precision is the key factor for success and will influence the functional response through biomechanics, yielding an aesthetic result. Psychological factors should also be included in this pre-operative evaluation.

Recreating a tissue environment in favour of the realisation of an aesthetic implant prosthesis may sometimes require several reconstructive surgeries.

The evaluation of the anatomical context before starting an implant treatment is very important and will allow the practitioner to have an idea of the extent of the necessary reconstructions.

To help the clinician in their assessment process—with the aim of identifying treatment possibilities, including aesthetic and functional objectives, as well as treatment limits—a classification was published by Dr. Palacci and Dr. Ericsson [4].

P. Palacci (✉)
Branemark Osseointegration Center Marseile, Marseille, France
e-mail: patrick@palacci.com



C. Barclay (ed.), *Oral Implantology: Assessment to Maintenance*, BDJ Clinician's Guides, https://doi.org/10.1007/978-3-031-55241-0_5

## 5.2 Classification

The Palacci–Ericsson classification is based on the amount of vertical and horizontal loss of hard and soft tissues. It divides the implant sites into four classes:

**Vertical Loss**

- Class I: Intact or slightly reduced papillae. (Fig. 5.1)
- Class II: Limited loss of papillae (less than 50%). (Fig. 5.2)
- Class III: Severe loss of papillae (more than 50%). (Fig. 5.3)
- Class IV: Absence of papillae (edentulous ridge). (Fig. 5.4)

**Horizontal Loss**

- Class A: Intact or slightly reduced buccal tissues. (Fig. 5.5)
- Class B: Limited loss of buccal tissues. (Fig. 5.6)
- Class C: Severe loss of buccal tissues. (Fig. 5.7)
- Class D: Extreme loss of buccal tissue, often in combination with a limited amount of attached mucosa. (Fig. 5.8)

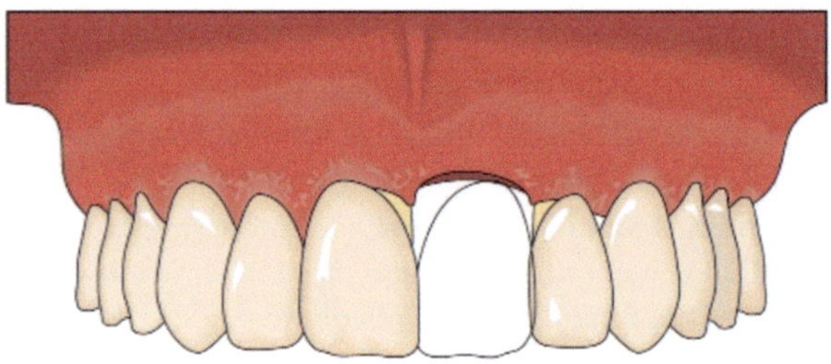

**Fig. 5.1** Class I: Intact or slightly reduced papillae

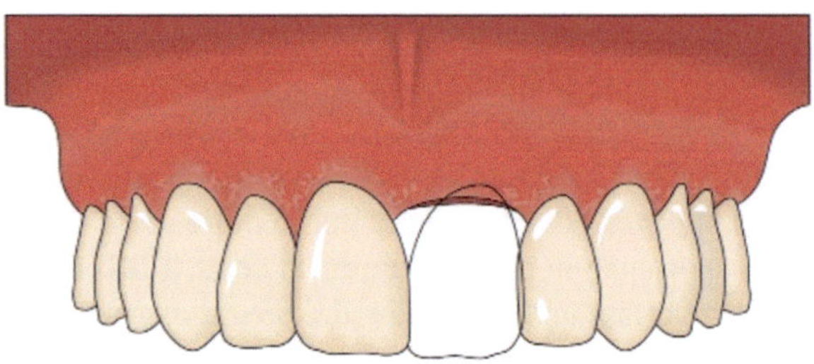

**Fig. 5.2** Class II: Limited loss of papillae (less than 50%)

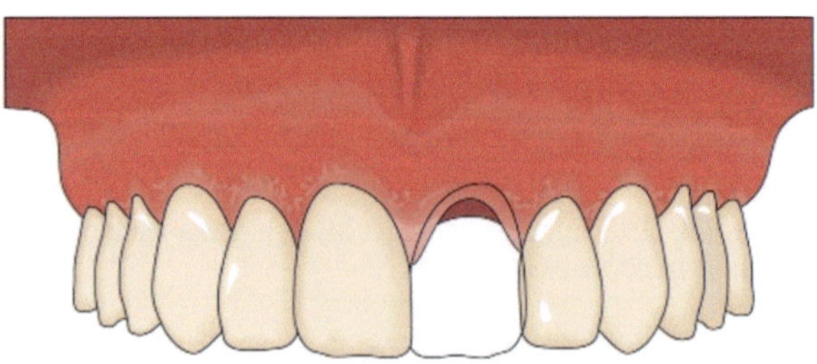

**Fig. 5.3** Class III: Severe loss of papillae (more than 50%)

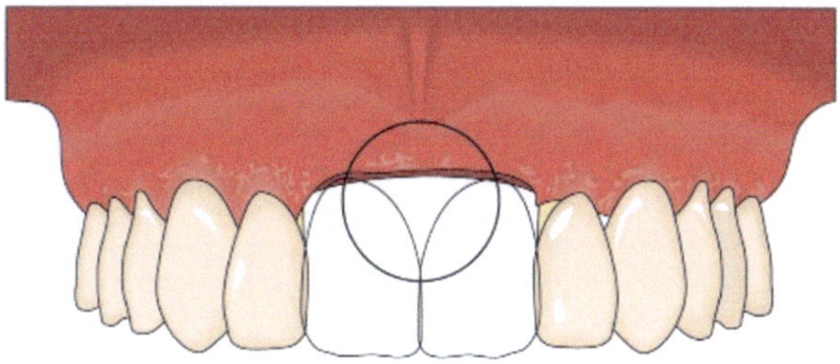

**Fig. 5.4** Class IV: Absence of papillae (edentulous ridge)

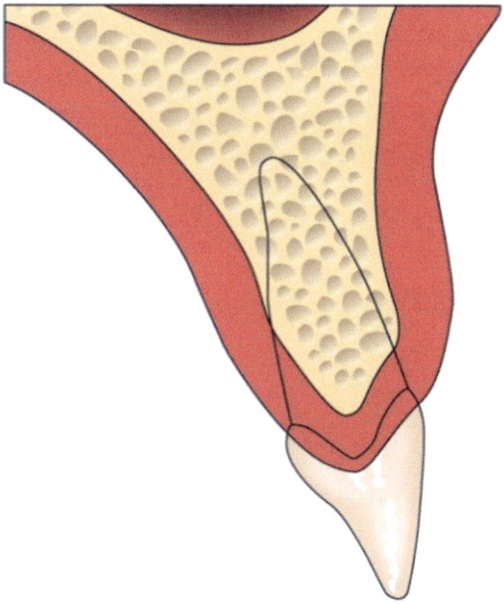

**Fig. 5.5** Class A: Intact or slightly reduced buccal tissues

Combinations of the different classes can co-exist, and each patient should be considered unique.

One should acknowledge that it is not possible to go directly from class IV to class II or from class III to class I in one surgery and realise that several additive procedures have to be performed to obtain the final optimal result.

Therefore, it is very important to identify the complexity of the case when we think about the treatment plan.

In some instances, the referring dentist, the surgeon and patient should realise that "restitution-ad-integrum" is not possible and that, in specific clinical situations, prosthetic tricks such as pink acrylic or porcelain may be needed to optimise the appearance.

Patients should be made aware of the aspects of the treatment before commencing.

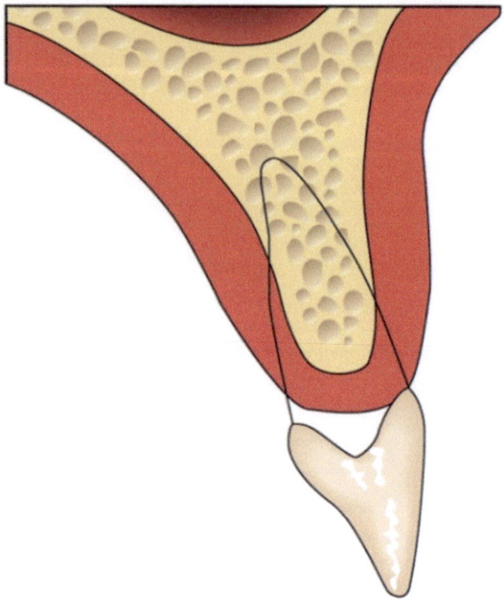

**Fig. 5.6** Class B: Limited loss of buccal tissues

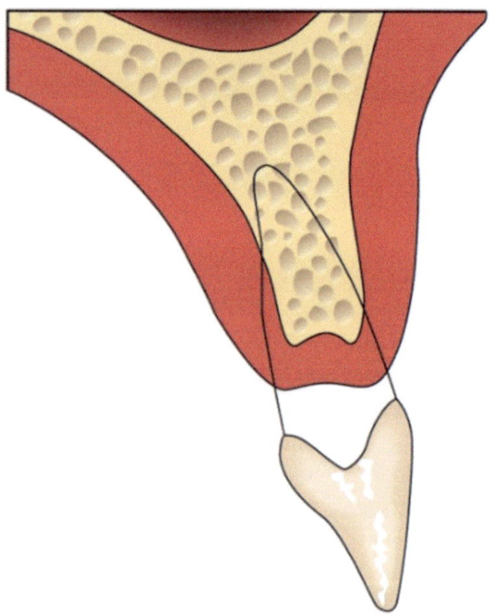

**Fig. 5.7** Class C: Severe loss of buccal tissues

This highlights the need for careful analysis of the case at the start of treatment, which involves evaluating the smile line, lip mobility and the aesthetic needs of the patient.

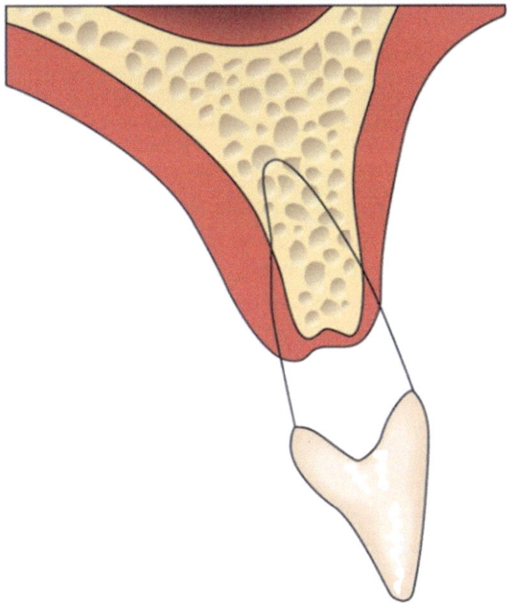

**Fig. 5.8** Class D: Extreme loss of buccal tissues, often in combination with a limited amount of attached mucosa

Only then will patients be able to understand the importance of additive surgeries influencing the time, expenses and morbidity of the overall treatment.

However, the surgeon should bear in mind a remark from PI Brånemark: "when possible one should avoid unnecessary advanced and complicated major grafting protocol".

## 5.3 Hard-Tissue Management

It is essential to ensure that a sufficient quantity of hard tissue is available in order to optimise implant positioning and stability. Different augmentation procedures are described to achieve this objective. Hard tissue may be added:

- Horizontally
- Vertically
- Both

Autogenous bone grafts (the patient's own bone), allograft (bone from the same species), xenograft (bone from a different species) or alloplastic materials (synthetic materials) may be used in block or particulate form, with or without resorbable or non-resorbable membranes to recreate the lost anatomy.

In general, hard-tissue augmentation is more predictable in horizontal than in vertical dimension due to a combination of factors such as blood supply and soft-tissue covering [1].

These surgical techniques should be performed by experienced surgeons because of the risk of complications.

However, one technique should be used by almost every implant surgeon: ridge preservation.

When extracting a tooth, we know that significant resorption in all dimensions will follow. Additive procedures will then be needed to recreate the lost tissues.

If, at the time of extraction, the practitioner is able to decontaminate the site and carefully compact a biomaterial such as collagenated xenograft (porcine material added with collagen, in this case—Osteobiol mp3 and by sticky xenograft (Osteobiol)), cover the site with a collagen membrane, optimal results may be achieved, avoiding complex additional procedures later on such as sinus lift.

This protocol, extremely useful and predictable, can be performed by any implantologist prior to implant placement as well as a general dentist at the time of extraction (Figs. 5.9, 5.10, 5.11, 5.12, and 5.13).

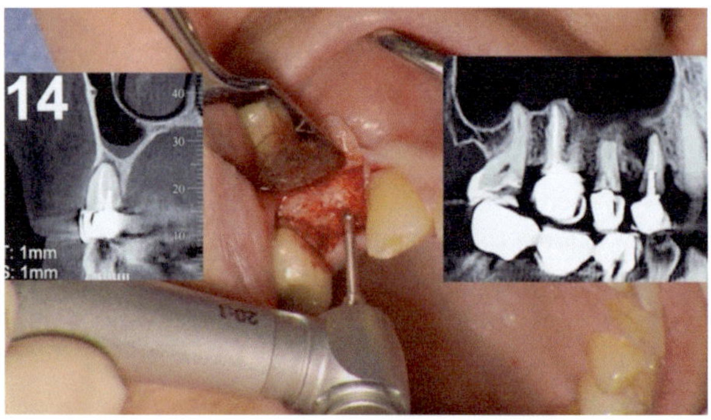


**Fig. 5.9** Extraction of 14 after curettage of the region and disinfection. Biomaterial (mp3 Osteobiol) is condensed

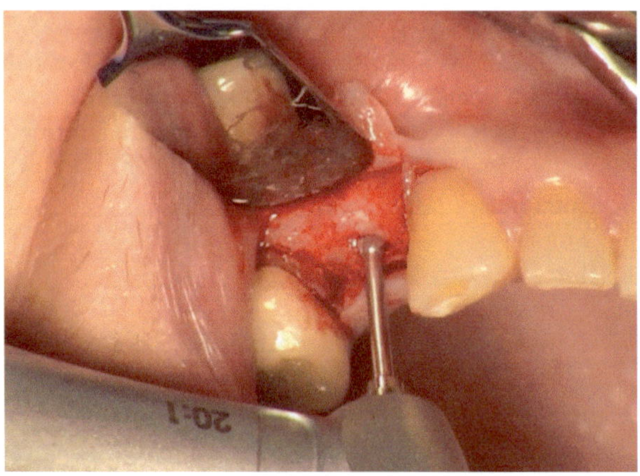

**Fig. 5.10** Three months later note the optimal bone reconstruction

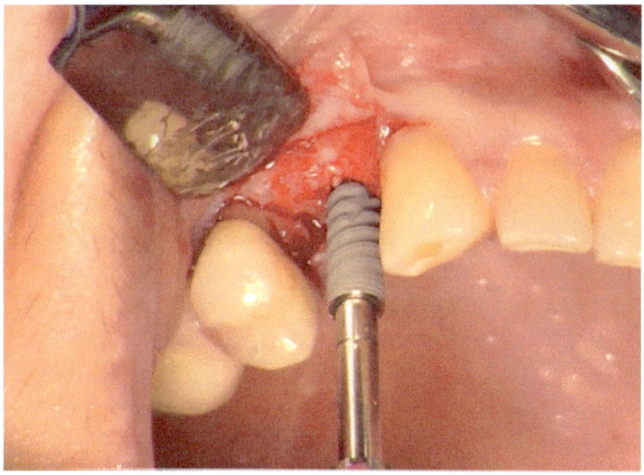

**Fig. 5.11** An implant is inserted (Nobel Active 3.5ø NobelBiocare)

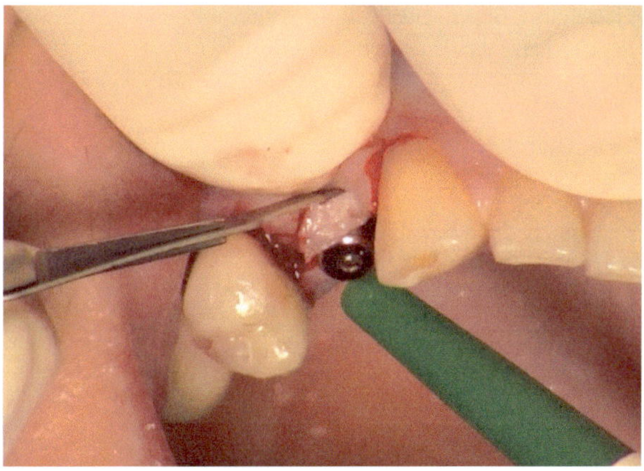

**Fig. 5.12** Papilla technique. Pedicle flaps are rotated from distal to mesial

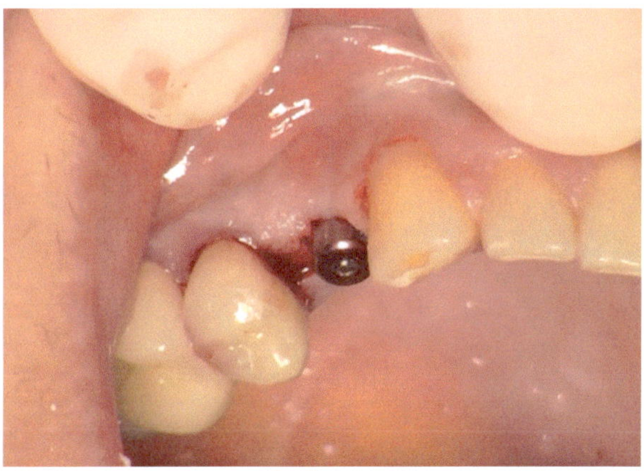

**Fig. 5.13** Optimal adaptation of the flap around the healing abutment

## 5.4 Soft-Tissue Management

Implant surgery can be performed using a one-stage or a two-stage procedure. Literature has shown no significant difference between the two options concerning the success rate [2].

All of the following techniques can be applied regardless of whether a one-stage or two-stage procedure is selected.

- In case of class 1A, the goal is to maintain and preserve the existing tissues.

In case of an extraction combined with an implant placement and immediate loading, one should focus on preserving the labial tissue and add, if necessary, connective tissue in order to recreate the coffin of dense connective tissue surrounding the abutment. No compression should be applied by a prosthesis in order to preserve the existing papillae (Figs. 5.14 and 5.15).

In case of an edentulous ridge with a dense connective tissue ridge, a tissue punch technique may be indicated.

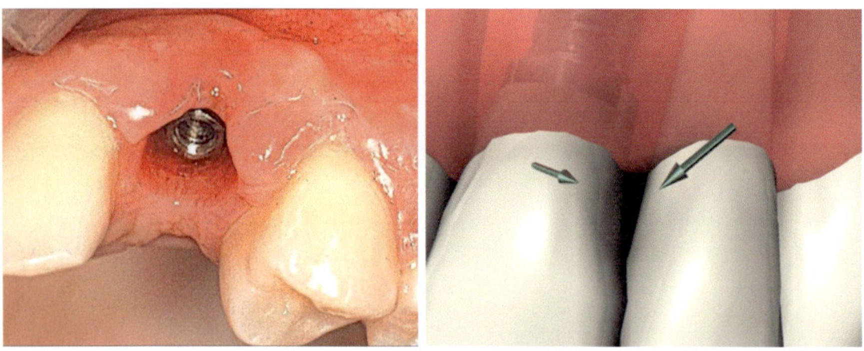

**Fig. 5.14** Implant placed in position 23. Implant positioning is the key for success as soft tissue will grow by itself

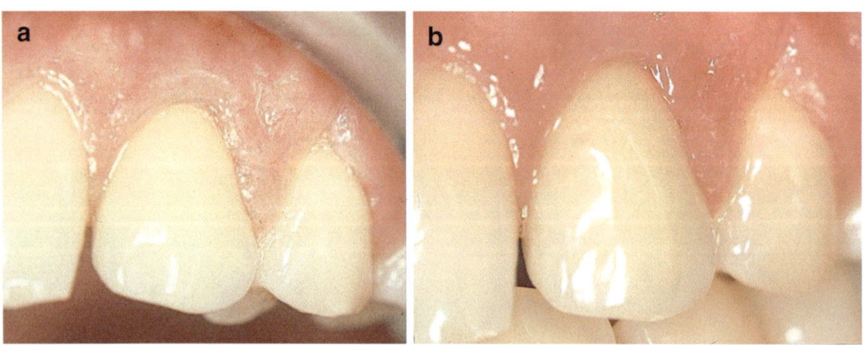



**Fig. 5.15** (**a**) 1-year follow-up (**b**) 14-year follow-up

In all other clinical situations, a crestal incision, followed by elevation of a full-thickness flap will be an appropriate option as a 2-mm growth of soft issue can be expected from the initial situation between the adjacent teeth and implant or between implants once the final restoration is placed [3].

- In case of a class II B with a moderate horizontal resorption and a papilla loss superior to 50%, a specific technique is needed. The technique developed by Palacci (Palacci flap) is certainly one of the most predictable techniques to be considered.

### 5.4.1 Loss of More Than 50% of the Papillae to Complete Loss of the Papillae

Bone is necessary to support a papilla and thus the height of any interdental papilla is related to the underlying bone level. So, in cases of severe bone loss, a bone graft should be performed prior to fixture installation, for which autogenous bone graft is still the gold standard. Ridge anatomy can also be significantly improved by connective tissue grafts [4–6].

The use of a bone graft will allow the clinician to:

- Create a hard-tissue support for implants and soft tissue/papillae
- Optimise implant positioning
- Optimise implant stability
- Optimise papilla reconstruction
- Optimise final aesthetics

### 5.4.2 Importance of Precise Implant Positioning

Implants should be adequately placed in all dimensions; however, specific attention should be given to the space between implants:

- If the space is too wide (over 8 mm from centre to centre), there will be too much space between the adjacent teeth and the papillae will not grow
- If the space is too narrow (less than 7 mm), there will not be enough blood supply for the peri-implant soft tissue and papillae will not grow well, resulting in poor oral hygiene and difficult maintenance, thereby compromising the long-term success of the implants (Figs. 5.16, 5.17, and 5.18)

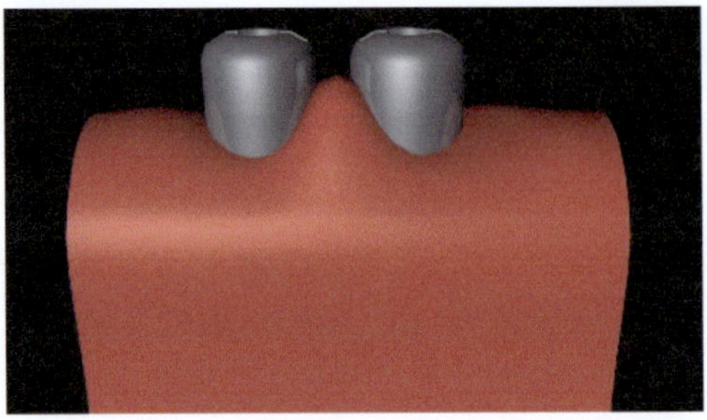

**Fig. 5.16** Optimal position of the implants (7–8 mm from centre to centre)

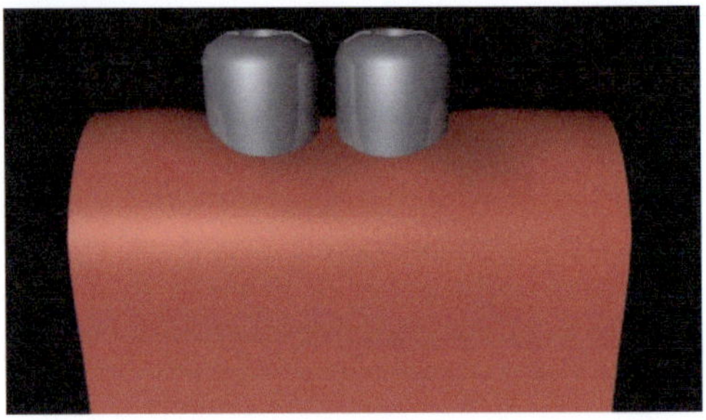

**Fig. 5.17** Less than 7 mm no papillae

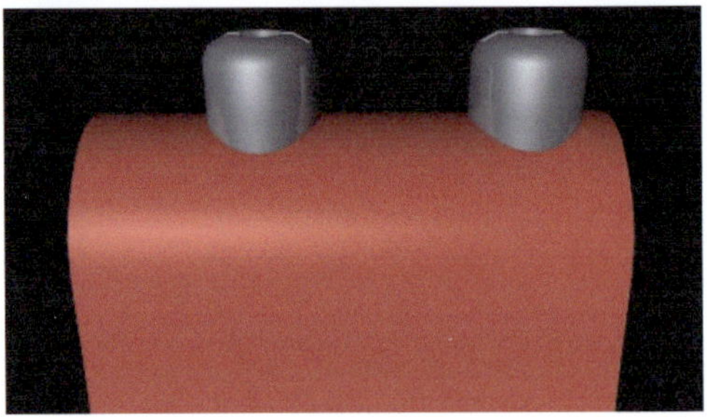

**Fig. 5.18** More than 8 mm no papillae

### 5.4.3 Surgical Reconstruction Technique to Recreate a Papilla-Like Formation Between Implants [7]

Careful manipulation of the peri-implant tissue may induce the required healing and the construction of soft-tissue architecture similar to the pre-morbid papillae. This manipulation can be performed at the time of fixture installation in the case of single-stage surgery or at the time of second-stage events.

A palatal incision allows the reflection of a full-thickness flap to the buccal aspect of the alveolar ridge, thereby increasing the volume on the buccal side of the implants. This tissue is stabilised by the healing abutments placed on top of the implants or the temporary crowns if an immediate prosthetic restoration is planned.

The excess labial tissue allows for dissection and rotation of pedicles:

- A semi-lunar incisor will recreate the scalloped shape of the soft tissue seen around the natural teeth.
- The pedicle of connective tissue (being perfectly vascularised) will fill the space between the abutments.
- The pleat created at the base of the rotated pedicle will be the base of the newly formed papilla (Figs. 5.19, 5.20, 5.21, 5.22, 5.23, 5.24, and 5.25).

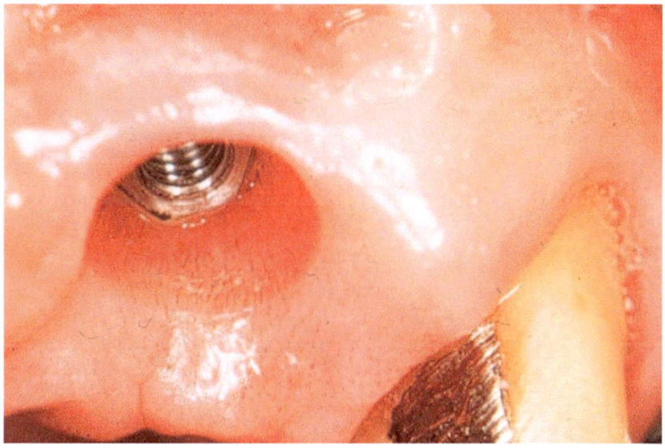

**Fig. 5.19** Papilla-like formation created using the papilla regeneration technique (Palacci)

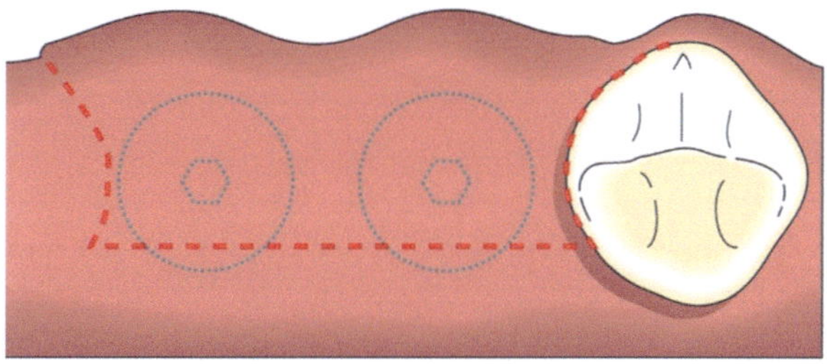

**Fig. 5.20** Schematic drawings illustrating the technique

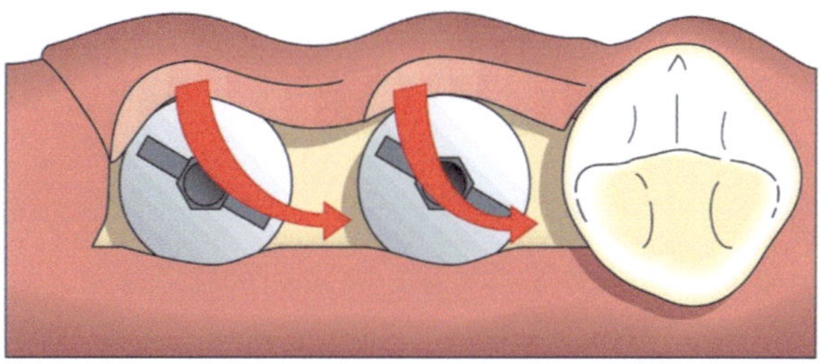

**Fig. 5.21** Schematic drawings illustrating the technique

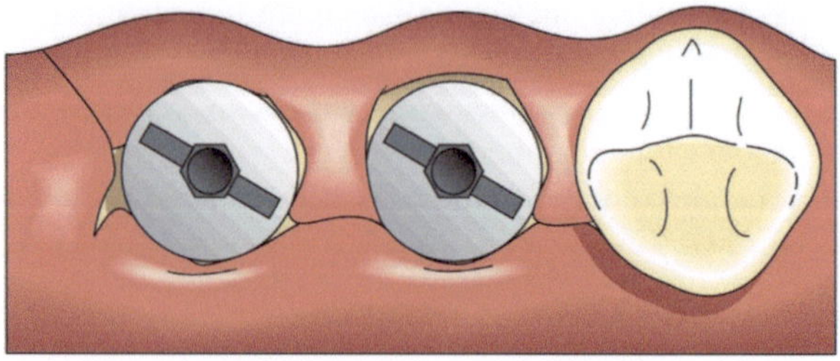

**Fig. 5.22** Schematic drawings illustrating the technique

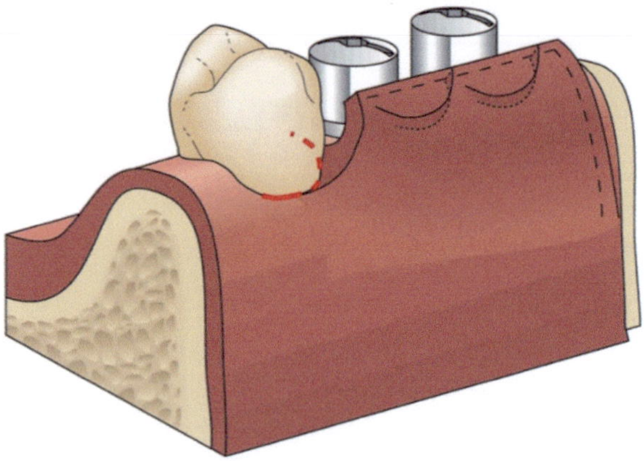

**Fig. 5.23** Schematic drawings illustrating the technique

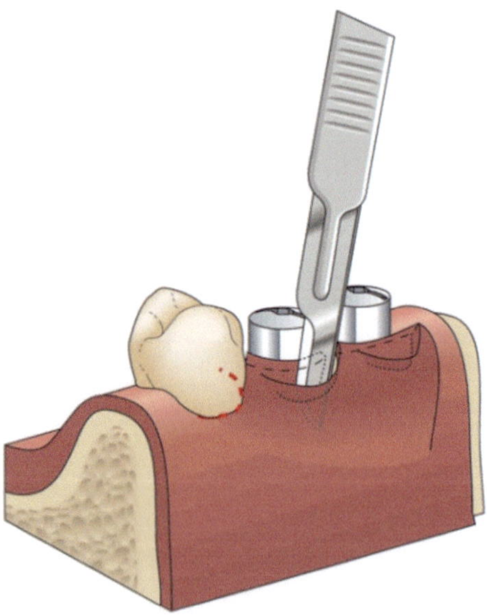

**Fig. 5.24** Schematic drawings illustrating the technique

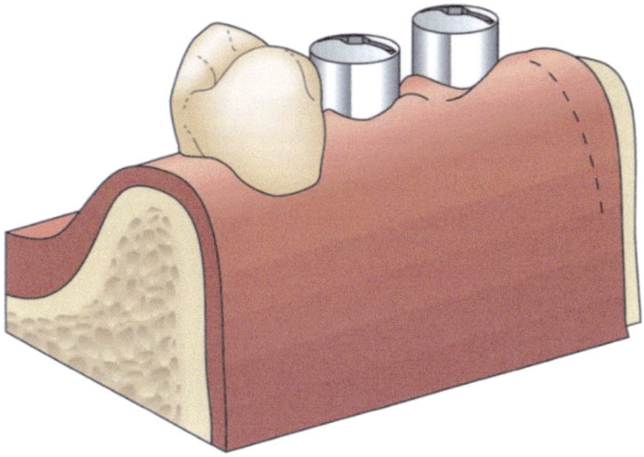

**Fig. 5.25** Schematic drawings illustrating the technique

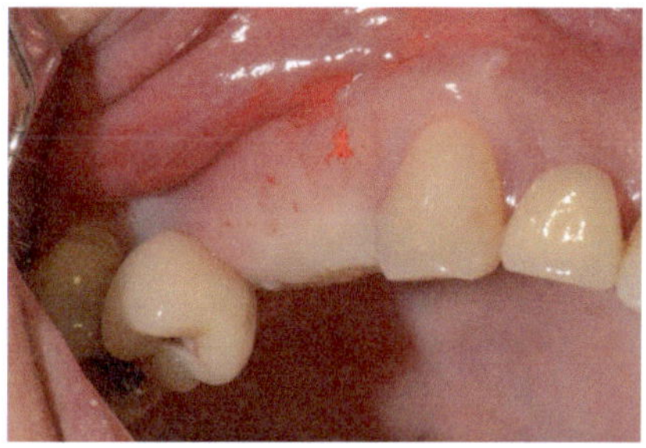

**Fig. 5.26** Pre-operative view of the implant site

There may be some variations of this technique:

- Pedicles can be rotated distally.
- Pedicles, more frequently created from a buccal flap, may be created from the palatal side, but one should note that the palatal tissues are difficult to manipulate.
- Combinations of different pedicles coming from various directions can be developed.

The technique to restore lost papillae involves the following general principles:

- Careful handling of the tissues in order to minimise trauma and maximise vascularisation.
- Bevelled incisions in the mobile flap should be carefully performed.
- The rotated pedicles should be tension-free (tension will result in ischaemia, loss of blood supply and loss of papillae) [8] (Figs. 5.26, 5.27, 5.28, 5.29, 5.30, and 5.31).

A mattress suture, starting on the labial side and going above the papillae to the palatal side, should provide a tight and firm connection of the pedicles to the supporting bone and abutments/crowns.

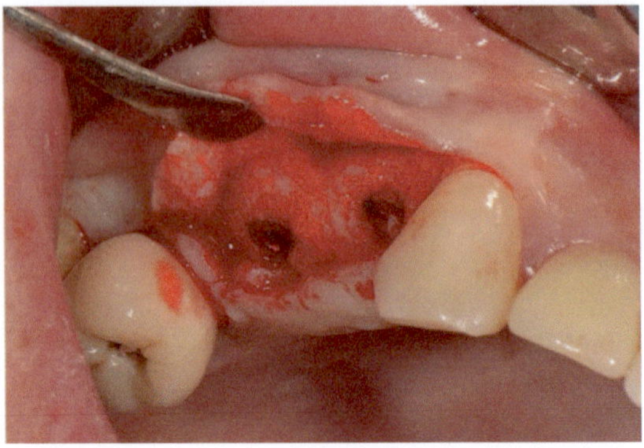

**Fig. 5.27** Raising flap and highlighting the two implants with cover-screws

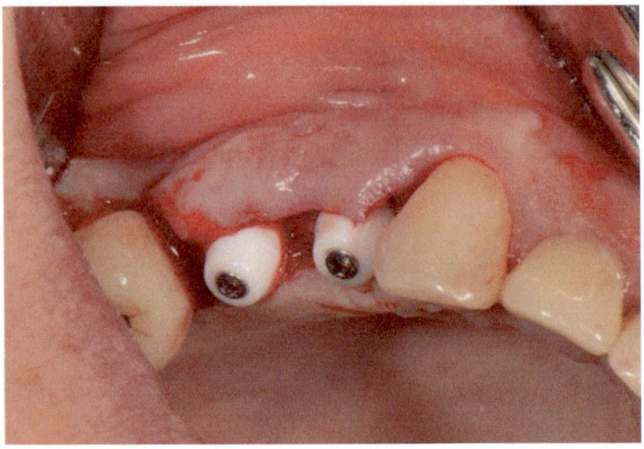

**Fig. 5.28** Placement of two multi-unit abutments with healing caps

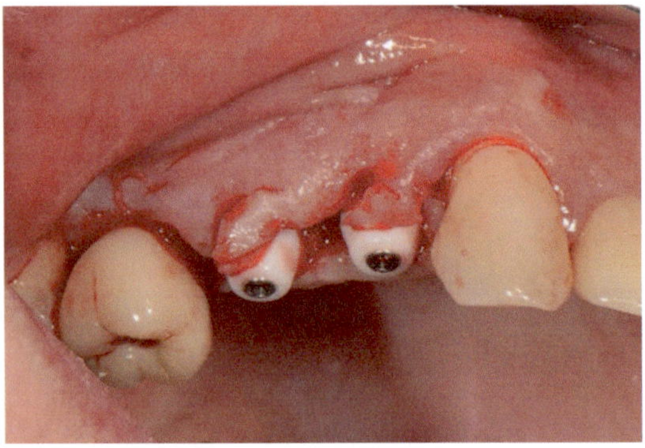

**Fig. 5.29** Semi-lunar bevelled incisions

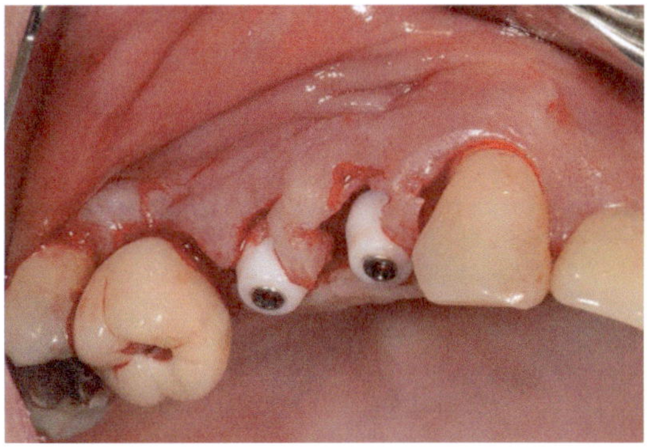

**Fig. 5.30** Semi-lunar incisions to recreate soft tissue in interproximal position

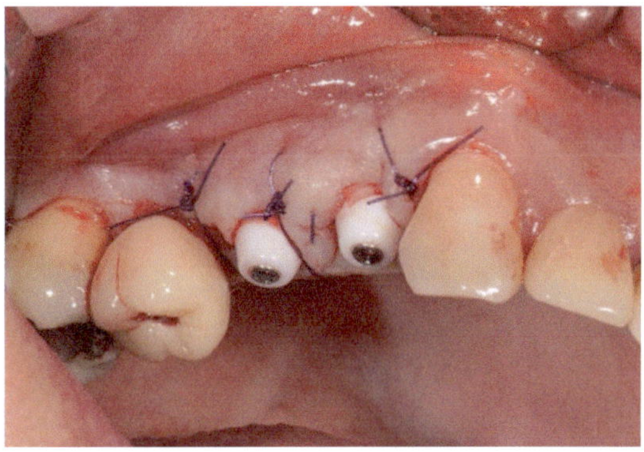

**Fig. 5.31** Rotated pedicles, tension-free mattress sutures providing a tight connection to the supporting bone and abutments

### 5.4.4 Single-Tooth Restoration

The same protocol can be used in case of single-tooth restorations; however, one should consider:

- The lack of space
- The lack of soft tissue
- The risk of ischemia
- The risk of cutting the papillae

A double-papillae technique can be used, but the risk of complications is high as two papillae have to be harvested from the labial flap.

Additive connective tissue grafts should be performed if necessary in order to be able to limit the pedicle to the mesial aspect (the more visible), and promote the mesial papilla (Figs. 5.32, 5.33, 5.34, 5.35, 5.36, 5.37, and 5.38).

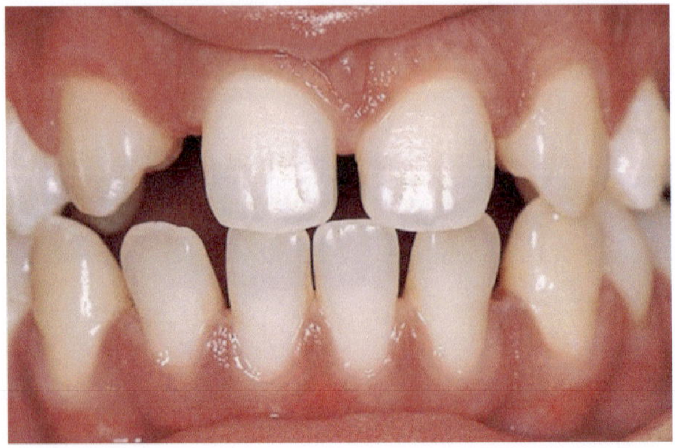

**Fig. 5.32** A 19-year-old female patient treated for lateral incisor anodontia

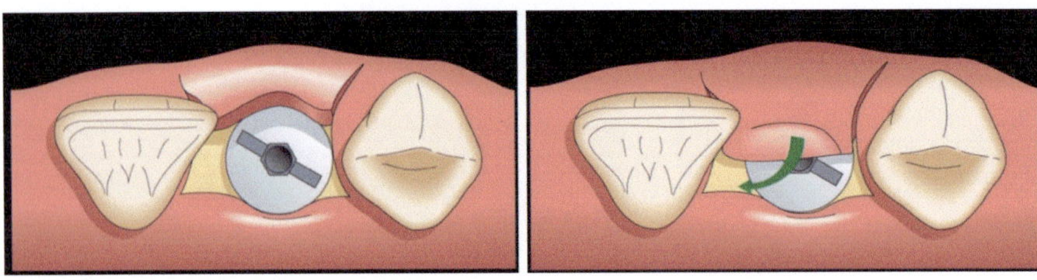

**Fig. 5.33** Schematic drawing: Papilla technique for single-tooth restoration

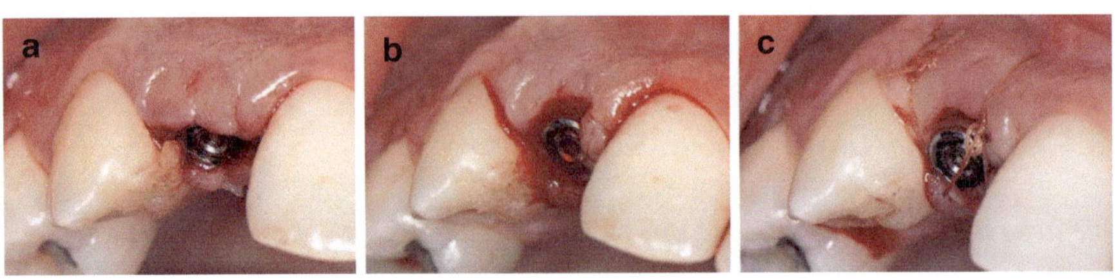


**Fig. 5.34** (**a**) Semi-lunar incision (**b**) Rotation (**c**) Suturing

**Fig. 5.35** Final case

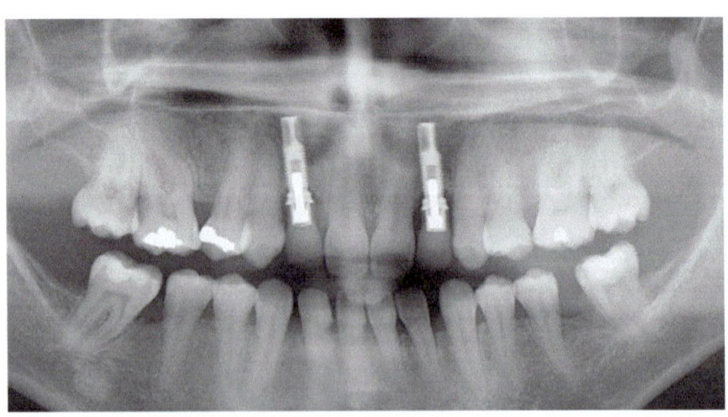

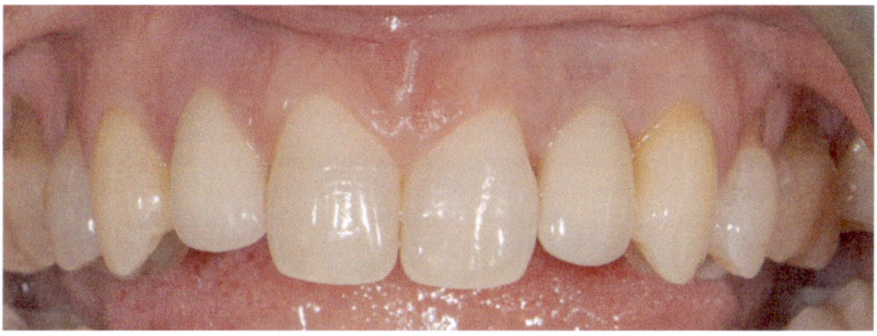

**Fig. 5.36** Aesthetic smile

**Fig. 5.37** Lip framework

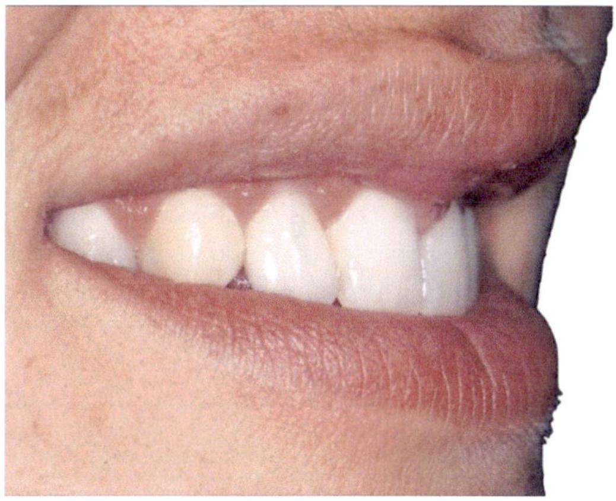

**Fig. 5.38** Gingival scaffold

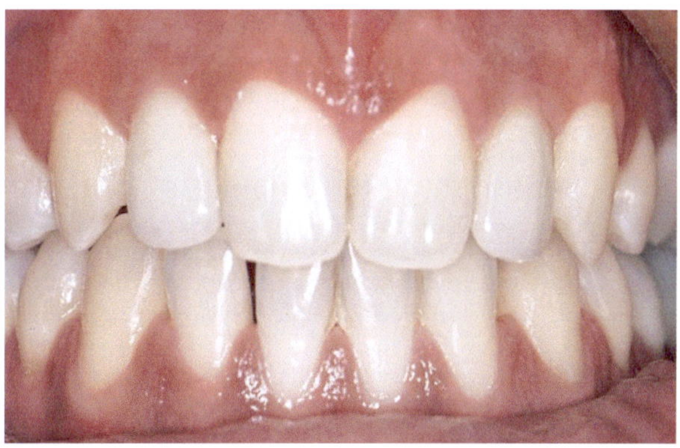

This technique can be considered as a soft-tissue plastic procedure. It obeys all the principles guiding any plastic surgery, i.e.:

- Respect of the blood supply
- Precise incisions
- Careful use of releasing incisions
- Perfect/optimal adaptation of the flaps
- Control of tissue tensions
- Precise suturing technique
- Use of sharp and selected instruments [9, 10]

## 5.5 Conclusion

The recreation of normal alveolar contour is paramount to aesthetic success. Restoration of the interproximal papillae is one of the last frontiers to be addressed in aesthetics of the anterior implant restorations.

Natural soft-tissue contour, thickness and colour are the requisites for maximising aesthetics of the anterior maxilla implant restorations. The aforementioned surgical principles and techniques, when carefully applied, allow the clinicians to obtain predictable, functional and aesthetically pleasing results.

## References

1. Moghadam HG. Vertical and horizontal bone augmentation with the intraoral autogenous J-graft. Implant Dent. 2009;18(3):230–8.
2. Gheisari R, Eatemadi H, Alavian A. Comparison of the marginal bone loss in one-stage versus two-stage implant surgery. J Dent (Shiraz). 2017;18(4):272–6.
3. Dimension of the periimplant mucosa. Biological width revisited – PubMed [Internet]. [cité 11 avr 2021]. https://pubmed.ncbi.nlm.nih.gov/8915028/
4. Palacci P, Ericsson I. Esthetic implant dentistry: soft and hard tissue management. Undefined [Internet]. 2001 [cité 11 avr 2021]. http://paper/Esthetic-Implant-Dentistry%3A-Soft-and-Hard-Tissue-Palacci-Ericsson/141fdf8c25078f9bab247d4b5bb4ebfd7721a92f
5. Optimal implant positioning & soft tissue management for the branemark system [Internet]. [cité 11 avr 2021]. http://www.quintpub.com/display_detail.php3?psku=B3083#.YHL9pT868uU
6. Palacci P, Nowzari H. Soft tissue enhancement around dental implants. Periodontol 2000. 2008;47(1):113–32.
7. The osseointegration book: from calvarium to calcaneus [Internet]. [cité 11 avr 2021]. http://www.quintpub.com/display_detail.php3?psku=B9018#.YHL-Bj868uU
8. Pontoriero R, Carnevale G. Surgical crown lengthening: a 12-month clinical wound healing study. J Periodontol. 2001;72(7):841–8.
9. Griffin TJ, Cheung WS, Zavras AI, Damoulis PD. Postoperative complications following gingival augmentation procedures. J Periodontol. 2006;77(12):2070–9.
10. Israelson H, Plemons JM. Dental implants, regenerative techniques, and periodontal plastic surgery to restore maxillary anterior esthetics. Int J Oral Maxillofac Implants. 1993;8(5):555–61.

# Restorative Options

# 6

Julian Satterthwaite

When considering the potential options available to restore implants, the interplay between planning and restoration cannot be underestimated. Placing one (or more) implants with a surgically driven mindset without a predetermined restorative plan is doomed to result in a sub-optimal functional and aesthetic outcome. Thus, surgical planning requires an understanding of restorative solutions and basic prosthodontic principles and concepts.

A key concept in determining restorative possibilities is that of the *prosthetic envelope*. In essence, the prosthetic envelope describes the space available for the provision of the restoration. This is effectively the distance from implant fixture head to opposing dentition, incorporating the interocclusal space. The prosthetic envelope must be considered three-dimensionally: as the complexity of restoration increases, the three-dimensional bulk of this restoration will also increase, impacting on function and phonetics as well as aesthetics.

Despite the critical nature and relative simplicity of this concept, its importance is too-often overlooked. This is particularly apparent in patients who present with concomitant tooth wear and tooth loss, where the loss of occlusal-vertical dimension (OVD) and subsequent reduction in space is poorly recognised. In some cases, a lack of available space might preclude the ability to place and restore an implant at all.

The space available in the prosthetic envelope (or considered another way, the tissues needing to be replaced) will directly impact the choice of type of restoration, including the abutment, mesostructure (sometimes referred to as a 'primary' superstructure), and superstructure, whilst also affecting the implant positioning and planning. There is clearly an interplay with resorptive patterns, prosthetic envelope, and the type/classification of restoration. The classic classification for prosthetic options was described by Misch [1] as below:

J. Satterthwaite (✉)
Restorative Dentistry, Division of Dentistry, School of Medical Sciences, The University of Manchester, Manchester, UK
e-mail: julian.satterthwaite@manchester.ac.uk



C. Barclay (ed.), *Oral Implantology: Assessment to Maintenance*, BDJ Clinician's Guides, https://doi.org/10.1007/978-3-031-55241-0_6

- FP-1
  - Fixed prosthesis; replaces only the crown; looks like a natural tooth.
- FP-2
  - Fixed prosthesis; replaces the crown and a portion of the root;
  - crown contour appears normal in the occlusal half but is elongated or hypercontoured in the gingival half.
- FP-3
  - Fixed prosthesis; replaces missing crowns and gingival colour and portion of the edentulous site
- RP-4
  - Removable prosthesis; typically an overdenture supported completely by implants
- RP-5
  - Removable prosthesis; typically an overdenture supported by soft tissue and implant

## 6.1 Restorative Options for Single Units (FP-1 & FP-2)

The resorptive processes and prosthetic envelope for FP-1 and FP-2 cases are relatively easy to visualise. In such cases, bone resorption is usually limited or minimal, and where only single teeth or a few teeth are to be replaced, the prosthetic envelope is readily identifiable. Despite this simplicity, there are still a variety of options available to retain the prosthesis.

### 6.1.1 Preformed Abutment and Cemented Crown

The simplest option entails placing a transmucosal abutment onto the implant fixture and then cementing a crown onto this abutment. An important distinction here is that the abutment may be preformed ('stock') or customised. Early preformed abutments (as well as many current versions) are often basic in shape with a margin at a continuous/even level (Fig. 6.1), sometimes with a matching component onto which the crown is built.

Although stock abutments are convenient and easy to use and often have excellent retention of the crown (due to walls that are parallel or with limited taper) they have some disadvantages. Following cementation it is difficult to ensure that all cement is removed from difficult to access sub-gingival margins; furthermore, stock abutments tend to have a 'narrow' restorative platform at a relatively coronal aspect leading to an unfavourable emergence profile and poor soft-tissue support. Typically, the abutments will be titanium and the crown would be porcelain-fused-to-metal (PFM).

Preformed abutments that are designed to be modified in the laboratory are also available, either as a 'blank' or with some limited existing sculpting such that they

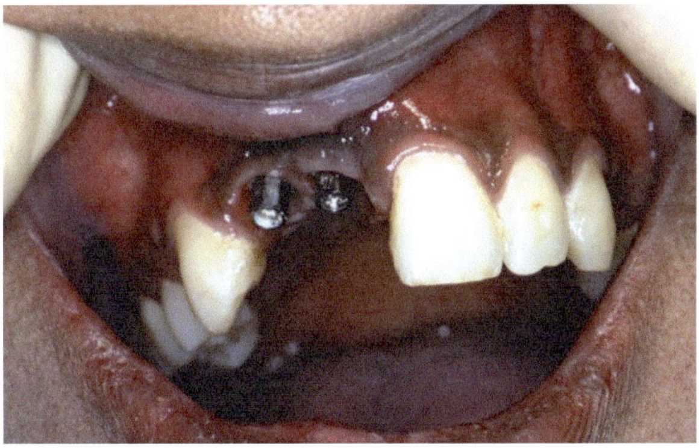

**Fig. 6.1** Stock abutments (CeraOne)—note continuous level and relatively deep subgingival margin

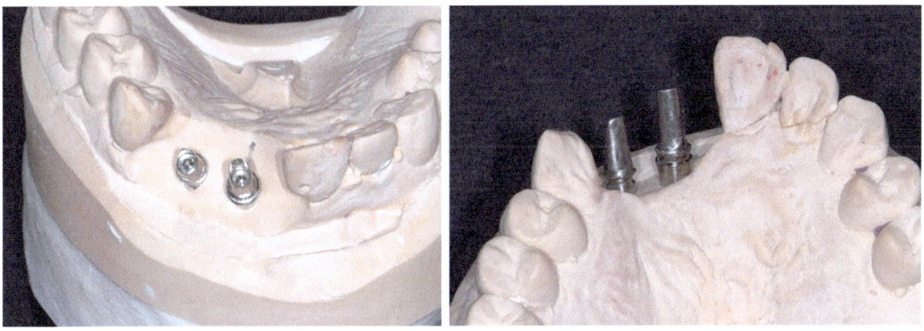

**Fig. 6.2** Narrow platform and limited anatomy with modified abutments

have some contour of the margins, although this remains fairly basic (Fig. 6.2). Although offering some advantages compared to simple stock abutments, they have the same disadvantages albeit to a lesser degree.

### 6.1.2 Fully Custom Abutment

Fully custom abutments are designed alongside the definitive crown restoration, without relying on stock components. Early fully custom abutments were constructed by casting gold or a bonding alloy onto a preformed 'precision fit' component, termed a 'UCLA- abutment' [2], typically then restored with a PFM crown. However, this technique is technically demanding, time-consuming and thus relatively expensive. The widespread adoption of CAD/CAM technology has transformed the up-take of fully custom abutments. These offer the simplicity of a cement-retained restoration with precision fit, good anatomical contour and emergence profile, and good soft-tissue support. Figure 6.3 demonstrates how fully custom abutments are more appropriately shaped, thus reducing the excess bulk of the overlying crown and facilitating easier cement clean up.

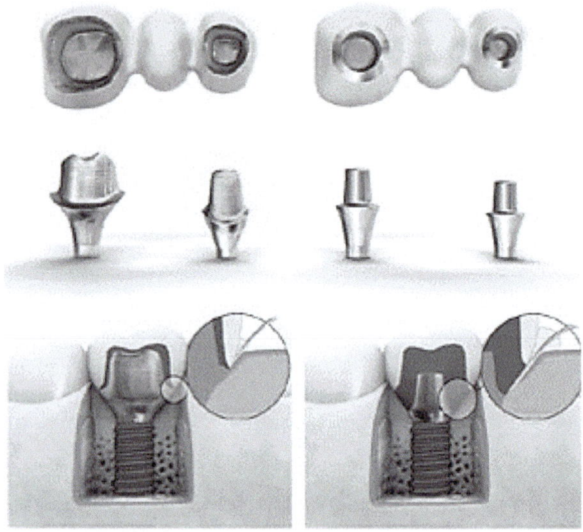

**Fig. 6.3** Diagram to highlight differences between custom and stock abutment. Note higher cementation margin on custom abutment and improved anatomical form

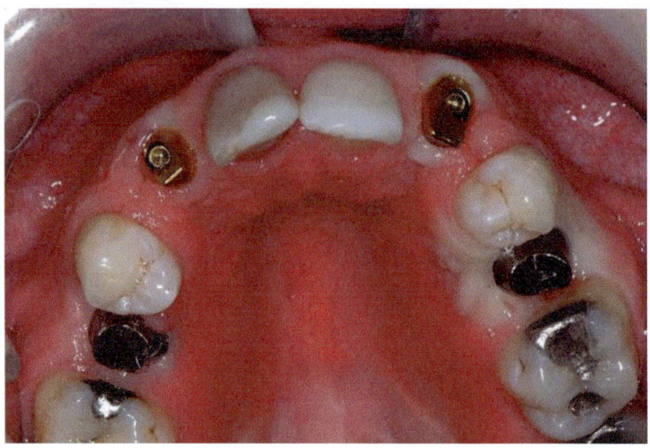

**Fig. 6.4** FP-1 prosthesis: implant-retained crowns UR2, UL2 (custom titanium abutments anodised)

Commonly, fully custom abutments are milled from titanium (often anodised with a gold hue to avoid a grey 'shine through' with thin gingival tissues: Fig. 6.4) or zirconia (Fig. 6.5), which although not as robust as titanium provides optimal aesthetics. Although crowns can be constructed with an opaque zirconia core that can mask an underlying metal abutment, typically a PFM crown tends to be provided where metal abutments are used (an example of PFM crowns for an FP-2 prosthesis is shown in Fig. 6.6), with all-ceramic crowns being provided where zirconia abutments are used.

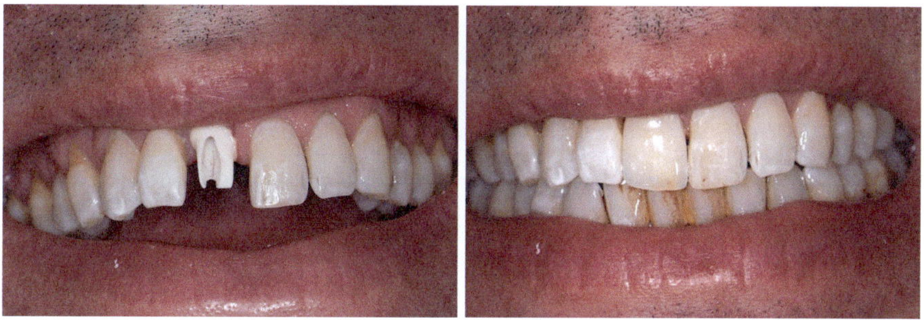

**Fig. 6.5** Example of FP-1 prosthesis: implant-retained crown UR1 (custom zirconia abutment and cemented crown)

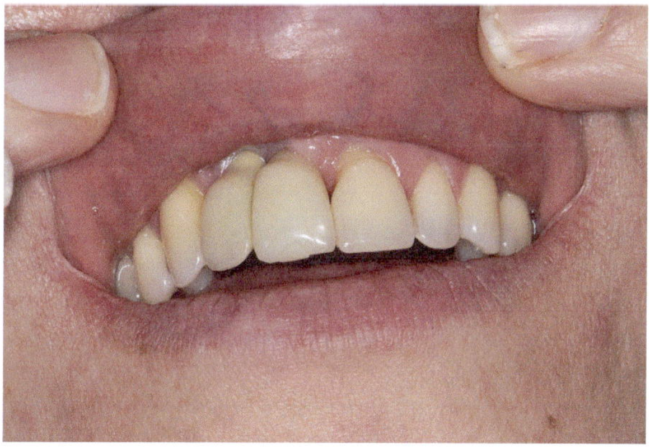

**Fig. 6.6** Example of FP-2 prosthesis: implant-retained crowns UR1 and UR2 also replacing a portion of the root (thankfully in this case a low lip-line hides the compromised aesthetics)

### 6.1.3 Screw-Retained Crown

Classically, screw-retained restorations involve placing an intermediate transmucosal abutment into the implant fixture, onto which the prosthesis is then attached with a screw (i.e. abutment level restoration). For a single unit, this is often not practical due to the narrow restorative platform at/near the gingival margin and thus for a screw-retained single crown it is more practicable to provide a single-piece solution whereby the crown is placed directly into the implant fixture and retained with a single screw (i.e., 'straight-to-fixture' with no separate intermediate abutment). In theory, an abutment level screw provides a 'weak point' coronal to the implant fixture and in the event of trauma (either acute or fatigue) of implant components the abutment level screw will fracture preferentially, sparing the implant fixture from irretrievable screw fragments in the implant body; however, available studies suggest that complications of fixture level screw-retained restorations are no higher than cemented crowns [3, 4].

Straight-to-fixture implant-retained crowns offer the simplicity and retrievability of screw retention with improved emergence profile (developed over a greater distance) and need less space due to lack of an intermediate abutment. Additionally, the lack of a transmucosal abutment may allow for a more cost-effective solution. As with all screw-retained restorations there are potential drawbacks of increased bulk to accommodate the screw-access channel (especially when used for anterior crowns) and reduction in control over occlusal contacts (due to the screw-access hole), although these are usually minor considerations.

### 6.1.4 'Screwmentable' and Hybrid Abutments

A potential draw-back of straight-to-fixture crowns is the difficulty in construction. Casting of fixture level components using traditional lost wax methods is not sufficiently precise and for a precision fit at the restoration: implant interface, a prefabricated component or a milled component is required. Construction of fully custom abutments using prefabricated components traditionally requires a cast-to approach (similar to the UCLA-type abutment described above) and is technically demanding and time-consuming, although in a similar manner solutions are now available whereby a zirconia abutment may be mechanically retained onto a prefabricated titanium base. However, for some implant systems, there are limited prefabricated options available and technicians often rely on third-party solutions, which may have implications on accuracy of fit [5] and manufacturer warranties.

A fairly recent development has been to provide a restoration that is constructed in two pieces yet delivered into the implant in a single piece. In essence this is similar to providing a custom abutment and cemented crown, but with the crown being formed to maintain a screw-access hole, and the abutment and crown being joined extra-orally. The two pieces are thus cemented in 'ideal' conditions and excess residual cement is not a problem: this provides a single-piece screw-retained restoration (sometimes referred to as 'screwmentable'). In many cases, it is possible to have a smaller screw-access hole, sometimes combined with a 'captive' screw. Although this approach has some significant advantages, the variation of construction approaches by different manufacturers can be confusing. It is also worth noting that current evidence base for their use, although promising, is relatively limited [6].

A potential problem where 'hybrid' systems are used (either where zirconia is mechanically attached to a titanium precision fitting element, or where abutment and crown are cemented together extra-orally) is that some solutions present a deep and even level marginal interface (a problem with all stock abutments) that is more difficult for the patient or professional to keep clean compared to the more superficial margin associated with a fully custom abutment. Careful communication with the technician is required to optimise possible solutions.

### 6.1.5 Screw Angle Correction

In many cases, the surgical positioning of an implant and subsequent long axis is such that a screw-access hole would be unfavourably positioned, e.g., on the labial aspect. This is particularly the case in the anterior maxilla where the normal anatomy and natural resorption patterns are such that the bony ridge is often 'angled' relative to the intended axial plane of the crown, in such a case placing an implant within the normal bony contour results in the long axis of the implant being labially inclined, with a screw-access channel being on the labial aspect of the crown. In order to achieve screw retention of a crown, through the desired palatal aspect, it would thus be necessary to 'upright' the implant angulation compared to the presenting bony ridge. Often this is straightforward and presents no issues, however, in many cases to do this would entail grafting or guided bone regeneration apically.

When faced with this scenario, the traditionally choice has been to accept a cement-retained restoration or accept more complex surgery. However, this is now much less of an issue with the advent of screw angle correction (angulated screw access/channel). Manufacturers vary slightly but typically this allows for correction of the screw-access channel of 20–30° with the use of a hexalobular driver and corresponding screw (Fig. 6.7). The result is the ability to provide screw-retained restorations simply, even with off-axis implant placement.

It has been argued that off-axis placement of a restoration can lead to long-term problems with implant health and subsequent failure due to unfavourable loading of

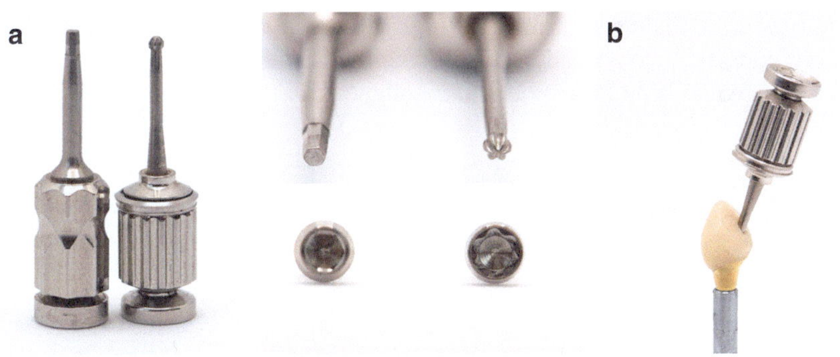


**Fig. 6.7** (**a**) Drivers and corresponding screws: standard hex, and hexalobular for angled screw access. (**b**) Screw angle correction allowing screw access at different angle to long axis of implant (avoiding incisal edge)

the implant away from its long axis, with concerns that this leads to stress concentration on crestal bone and possibly increased microgap formation between components, however these concerns do not appear to have materialised. A potential drawback of screw angle correction is the increased bulk/size required for the screw channel, but this is usually not an issue. An alternative approach, that obviously requires planning ahead, is to use a co-axis implant where the restorative interface of the implant head is not aligned with the fixture body and incorporates the 'angle correction'.

## 6.2 Considerations with Multiple Units (FP-1 & FP-2)

In essence, the methods of attachment for multiple units are no different to those outlined above for single units; however, there are several further considerations. The first relates to retrievability: quite simply, the larger the restoration, the higher the anticipated maintenance requirements, with higher incidences of fracture of the prosthesis, especially if full arch [7]. Although it is entirely possible to provide a cement-retained bridge that replaces multiple units, careful consideration should be given to the ease with which this can be removed if required. Extensive bridgework may be better split into smaller units (example shown in Fig. 6.8) as large span/cross-arch cement-retained bridges may prove challenging to remove.

Given the higher likelihood of having to remove a larger prosthesis for maintenance, it is much more sensible to consider screw retention in such cases. For screw retention, the choice is then needed as to whether to work at fixture level, with a straight-to-fixture bridge, or to work at abutment level with an intermediate 'multi-unit' abutment. The main issue with the former approach is that many implant systems have little tolerance for implant divergence when working at fixture level. It simply may not be physically possible to allow for seating of the prosthesis and provide a fixture level bridge on multiple implants which are divergent. The huge

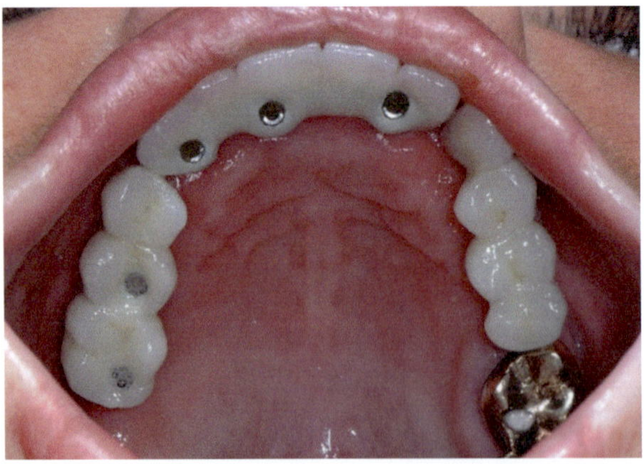

**Fig. 6.8** Full arch bridgework separated into three smaller units for ease of maintenance (mix of screw and cement-retained bridges)

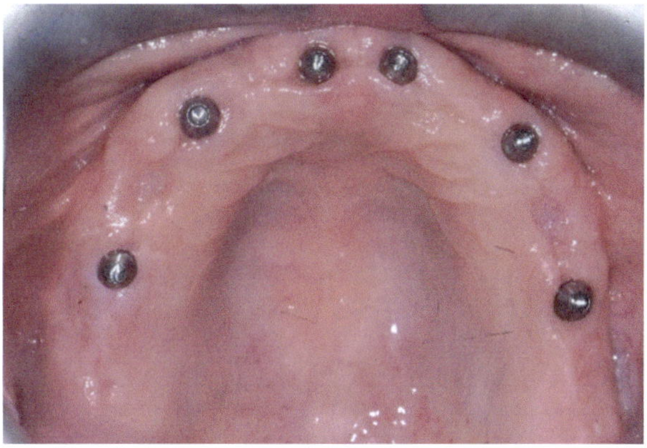

**Fig. 6.9** Multi-unit abutments in situ (Astra Tech EV uni-abutments) allowing for divergence of multiple implants

range of implant systems available, with variation in the amount of internal engagement from one system to another, can potentially make this a complex area. As a rule of thumb, provided the implant divergence is not great, multiple unit straight-to-fixture restoration on divergent implants is usually possible if the implant restorative connection is external or only minimally engages the internal aspect of the implant bodies. Where there is significant internal engagement (e.g., 'long cone' or parallel internal connections), then there is minimal scope for coping with even small degrees of divergence and an abutment level solution will be required (Fig. 6.9).

The potential drawbacks of multi-unit abutments are as per those of the stock abutments mentioned above—with larger bridges, careful planning of the three-dimensional position of the implants and choice of abutment height can minimise these drawbacks. Additionally, screw angle correction can be employed at abutment level to allow for better positioning of screw-access channels within the body of the prosthesis.

Traditionally, construction of an implant-retained bridge is PFM with a framework typically cast from bonding alloy and layered with porcelain. Typical alternative approaches now include zirconia frameworks, or milled metal frameworks (cobalt-chrome or titanium), again layered with porcelain. It is also possible to provide the teeth in composite as an alternative to ceramic which potentially has some advantages in relation to ease of maintenance/repair.

## 6.3 More Complex Restorations and FP-3

The categorisation of prostheses is less informative when considering more complex restorations. The FP-3 category covers a large range of possible prostheses and may be as simple as a small bridge that also replaces a small amount of soft tissue, ranging to a full arch restoration with significant 'gum work' to replicate the soft tissues. In general terms, the methods of construction and the potential means of

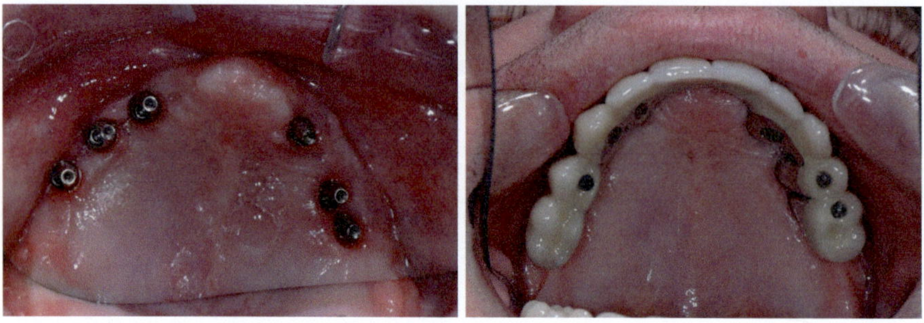

**Fig. 6.10** Example of angled multi-unit abutments (Astra Tx Angled uni-abutments) used to restore a full arch with challenging angulation of implants—note difference in axis of abutment screw (into implant body) and bridge screw

connection of the prosthesis and superstructure to the implants does not greatly differ from those outlined above for other multi-unit restorations; however, common key differences are more compromised surgical sites and larger prosthetic envelopes.

The more compromised surgical sites that are typical with situations where a large amount of soft-tissue requires replication often makes ideal implant positioning challenging and this often results in divergent implants. Thus, with larger prostheses, straight-to-fixture solutions become less likely with most being provided at abutment level. A further consideration is the axis of the implants and location of the screw-access holes: in many cases, a compromise might be required. For both situations, it is possible to use multi-unit abutments that are angled with the long axis of the prosthetic screw differing to the long axis of the abutment, providing angle correction typically in the range 15–30° (Fig. 6.10). There is a broad range of angled multi-unit abutments from different manufacturers, but common issues are limited angle correction possibilities, limited choice of abutment height and a tendency to be 'fiddly' to use. The widespread adoption of and ability to provide angulated screw access provides a significant benefit in many of these cases as an alternative to angled multi-unit abutments, however, they remain convenient for planned cases with angulated implants (e.g. 'All-on-four' approaches).

A more extensive loss of hard and soft-tissue results in a larger prosthetic envelope that dictates the need to prosthetically replace soft tissue as well as provide replacement teeth. In most cases, restorations would still be provided as a single piece superstructure, although the larger prosthetic envelope also allows additional space for more slightly more complex restorations that include a mesostructure. A broad range of options and materials for construction are available, but essentially these can be grouped into: layered frameworks (as described above) with pick porcelain or pick composite; an acrylic-wrapped framework; or mesostructures with separate teeth.

Where the prosthetic envelop is large and soft-tissue replacement is relatively extensive, an acrylic wrap with denture teeth is the simplest solution. A variety of sub-structure frameworks and materials including cast metals and also synthetics (e.g., PEEK) are possible, although milled titanium is perhaps the contemporary

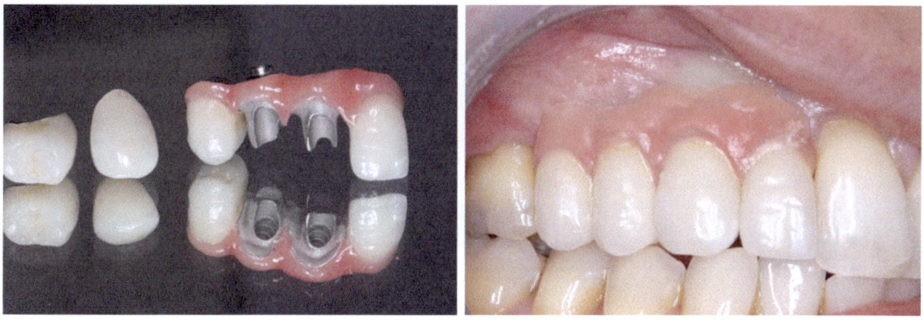

**Fig. 6.11** Example of a small FP3 bridge with mesostructure. (Images courtesy of Dr Liam McGrath)

'default'. These may be made either as a complete wrap with a 'hidden' framework, or with part of the external aspect, typically facing the tissues and/or lingually, being polished metal (e.g. a 'Montreal' bar). The large prosthetic envelope allows for multiple options for emergence of the screw-access, with the positioning of these being less critical than some other solutions, although compromises may still be required, perhaps with additional bulk of a prosthesis encroaching on lingual space.

Mesostructures may be designed with shaped extensions akin to individual crown preparations to which individual teeth may be attached. Proposed advantages of these are the ability to overcome difficult screw-access angulations (as an alternative to angled multi-unit abutments or angulated screw access) and provide optimal aesthetics with no screw-access holes being visible, yet with relatively easy access to the prosthetic screws if required. These are classically used for extensive bridges, but the technique can also be used in smaller cases (Fig. 6.11).

## 6.4 Restorative Options RP-4

The RP4 category appears straightforward: a removable prosthesis that is supported by implants, however, similar to FP3, there exists a wide variation in possible solutions within this category. The common factor for these prostheses is the use of a mesostructure of some description, with these broadly divided into: simple bar; beam and sleeve; or bar/beam with attachments.

### 6.4.1 Bar-Retained Dentures

A bar-retained denture is the easiest to visualise, and the most commonly provided. This comprises a bar that joins together the implants, with retentive clips ('riders') within the denture (Fig. 6.12). The denture will thus be almost fully implant-supported, allowing for much reduced tissue-coverage, favoured by many patients especially in the maxilla.

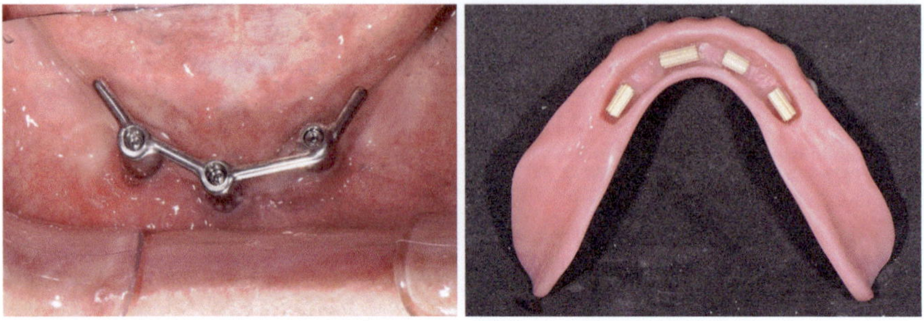

**Fig. 6.12** An implant-retained bar in situ with corresponding denture

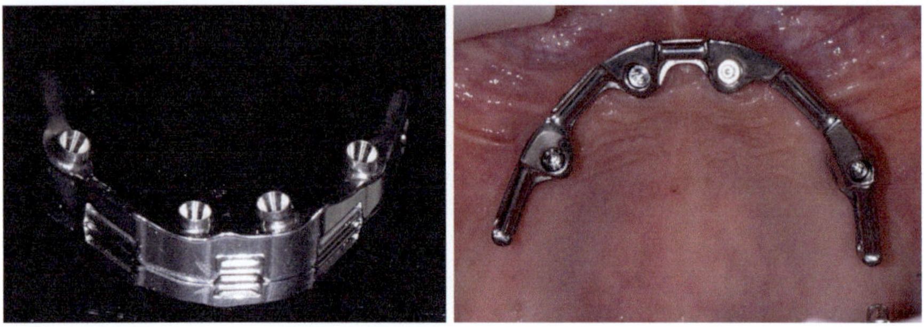

**Fig. 6.13** A preci-horix bar made at abutment level

There are several different designs of bar possible, with varying cross sections, the most common being simple Hader (round in cross section), modified Hader (with an extension towards the soft-tissue to provide additional strength and limit clip rotation), and preci-horix (rectangular cross section with milled retentive elements—Fig. 6.13). Dolder bars (usually egg-shaped in cross section, allowing more freedom of movement) are also available. Historically, bars were constructed from cast gold, but these are now almost universally milled CAD/CAM bars from titanium. Simple round bars have a low profile and are the most appropriate choice where the prosthetic envelope is relatively limited; there are slight advantages to shaped bars over simple round bars with proposed greater stability, although in many cases these are relatively small considerations. As with other attachments, there are a variety of different types of riders with these being simple gold clips (embedded in the denture base) or nylon inserts in a housing. Although the larger prosthetic envelope typically seen in patients requiring complete dentures provides some flexibility in implant positioning, the spacing between implants remains a key consideration when considering bar restorations. Should implants be placed too close together, there will be insufficient space to place a rider. There is some flexibility where gold clips are used (which can be shortened in length) but not when prefabricated housings and inserts are used.

As described earlier, it is possible to make bars at either fixture level or abutment level using a transmucosal multi-unit abutment. The same considerations regarding the internal connection and implant design are relevant regarding the ability to place at implant level with divergent implants, and thus abutment level bars are more common in the maxilla. The ability to provide an implant level connection may have some advantages where space is restricted. In cases where the prosthetic envelope is limited, then the use of a bar needs to be reconsidered and a simpler (and smaller) implant-retained (i.e., RP5) solution will be required: this should be identified at the planning stage.

### 6.4.2 Rigid Beams

It is also possible to provide an implant-supported removeable prosthesis with greater stability and retention with the use of differing mesostructures; in many cases, these can be considered 'hybrid' designs in that they have as much support and thus similar function as a fixed, whilst are removable with the advantages of cleansability and ease of reproducing missing soft tissues with a flange. The simplest such design is the use of a 'beam' on the implants and a matching 'sleeve' within the denture (Fig. 6.14). With this design, the retention relies on the precision friction fit of the sleeve against the beam. Constructing such a mesostructure from cast alloys (typically gold) requires a high level of skill, additionally the extra volume required to house these components requires a very large prosthetic envelope. Nonetheless, these systems allow for predictable restoration in challenging cases, including those with acquired or congenital anatomical defects (e.g., resection or clefts) where restoration would otherwise be a challenge. Despite the many advantages of CAD/CAM technology, this is one area where a milled framework and sleeve may not always provide the accuracy for retention through friction fit alone.

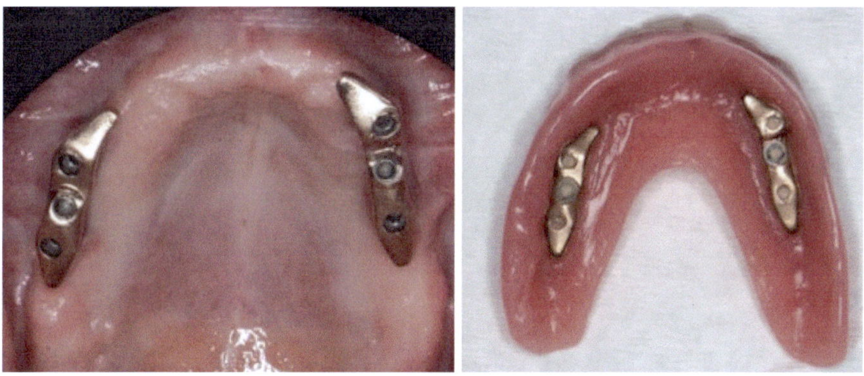

**Fig. 6.14** 13-year review of maxillary denture retained by bilateral milled beam and sleeve

A variation on the design above, which does lend itself to CAD/CAM is the use of a milled beam with supplementary attachments (Fig. 6.15). In its simplest form, this would be a milled beam without a matching sleeve, but with attachments such as a ball or locator placed into the beam (often the beam is milled with a screw thread into which a replaceable attachment is inserted). The denture is typically made without a corresponding sleeve, but with matrices for the attachments. Such designs are relatively common, however require a significant prosthetic envelope, rely primarily on the attachments for retention, and have reduced stability compared to the use of a sleeve due to the lack of intimate fit and reduced horizontal/rotational bracing.

The placement of attachments on a beam can overcome some issues with rider positioning if implant placement is not ideal and a large beam allows for good stability of a prosthesis although in many cases there is limited advantage in the use of these compared to simpler solutions such as preci-horix bar that requires a smaller volume. When used with a corresponding sleeve there is greater stability and the easier construction of a milled CAD/CAM beam over a handmade gold beam is attractive, although again, the prosthetic volume required should not be underestimated.

It is also possible to construct a beam and sleeve with retentive elements or a latch to provide fixation of the two components (Fig. 6.16), thus providing ultimate

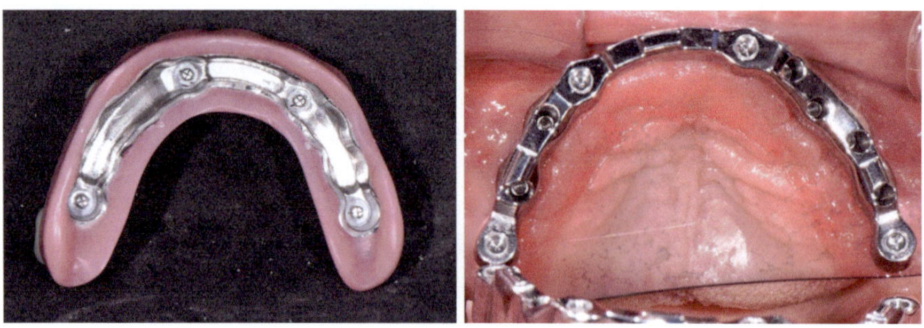

**Fig. 6.15** CAD/CAM titanium milled beam and sleeve with additional attachments

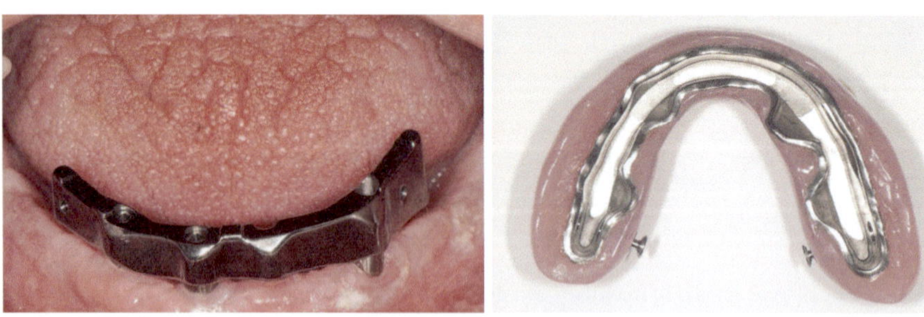

**Fig. 6.16** CAD/CAM telescopic restoration: mesostructure in situ and superstructure with latch attachments posteriorly

stability and retention of a removable prosthesis and a true 'hybrid' approach. Different manufacturers use different terminology such as '2-in-1' or 'telescopic': such systems require a considerable degree of manual dexterity of the patient for their removal and insertion.

## 6.5 Restorative Options RP-5

An implant-retained denture is the simplest prosthetic solution utilising implants, the denture being mostly mucosa-supported (tissue borne) but prevented from full displacement by being removably attached to implants. Given the lack of significant support from the implants, basic denture principles and full coverage of the denture bearing area is usually needed to provide the required tissue support and a degree of bracing. This is a key distinction when explaining the proposed outcome to patients, in that some movement of the denture is still likely, although satisfaction and quality of life with implant-retained dentures is much higher compared to conventional dentures [8, 9] and is generally seen as a standard of care [10, 11]. It is worth noting that although maintenance has been shown to be higher with the use of studs compared to bars [12], maintenance of stud-retained dentures is usually straightforward.

A variety of attachment systems exist, but in essence are all 'stud-type' with a shaped abutment attached to the implant and a matching retentive element housed within the denture. The two most common systems are ball-type attachments and locators (Fig. 6.17).

To a large degree, the choice of locator vs ball is personal, though the available space within the prosthetic envelope may dictate which approach is used. Locator-type abutments tend to have a lower profile than ball attachments, but a larger diameter. Female inserts for locators comprise a metal housing with a resilient nylon insert that provide retention and are available in differing strengths. 'Classic' locators have a tendency to trap debris within the abutment, although newer designs (e.g., R-Tx) have less of an issue in this respect.

Ball abutments are fairly universal in design, although diameters vary between different manufacturers. The female components vary and may be simply gold-leaf attachments processed into the denture, nylon inserts in a housing (e.g., Clix), or metal retentive elements within a housing (e.g., Dalbo Plus): it is axiomatic to state that removable elements within a housing are far easier to maintain and replace than

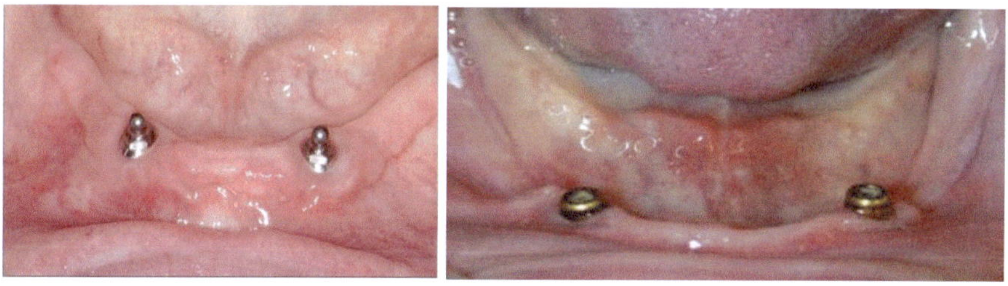

**Fig. 6.17** Examples of ball-type and locator abutments

those that are processed into the denture. With either type of abutment, ideally the height of abutments should be chosen such that they are in line with the occlusal plane, not necessarily an even height above the soft tissues.

In general terms, implants for stud attachments need to be parallel, although the use of nylon inserts allows for a little leeway in this regard, and locators inserts stated to allow up to 40° of misalignment are also available: abutments with angle correction are also available from some manufacturers.

The most common use of studs to retain a denture is for a mandibular denture retained by two studs. It is possible to use an additional number of implants for increased retention and stability although it tends to be more difficult to achieve parallelism for multiple implants which is necessary to allow even, simultaneous engagement of multiple studs. In situations where it is felt that greater retention and stability is required, it may be wiser to consider a bar instead. Conventionally, implants placed in the maxilla are recommended to be splinted, and thus, de-facto, the use of studs would not be recommended. There have, however, been various reports of successful use of individual implants with studs for maxillary dentures, although evidence remains limited [13]. In any event, the practicalities of achieving near-parallel placement of multiple implants in the maxilla often precludes the use of studs, although some implant systems now allow for angled attachments where the retentive element is at a different angle to the long axis of the implant (similar to angled multi-unit abutments).

## References

1. Misch CE. Bone classification training keys. Dent Today. 1989;8:39–44.
2. Lewis S, Beumer J 3rd, Hornburg W, Moy P. The "UCLA" abutment. Int J Oral Maxillofac Implants. 1988;3:183–9.
3. Wolfart S, Rittich A, Groß K, Hartkamp O, von der Stück A, Raith S, Reich S. Cemented versus screw-retained posterior implant-supported single crowns: a 24-month randomized controlled clinical trial. Clin Oral Implants Res. 2021;32:1484–95. https://doi.org/10.1111/clr.13849.
4. Lamperti ST, Wolleb K, Hämmerle CHF, et al. Cemented versus screw-retained zirconia-based single-implant restorations: 5-year results of a randomized controlled clinical trial. Clin Oral Implants Res. 2022;33(4):353–61. https://doi.org/10.1111/clr.13895. PMID: 35051314.
5. Rizvi N, Alyahya Y, Rizvi A, Narvekar U, Petridis H. Accuracy of original vs. non-original abutments using various connection geometries for single unit restorations: a systematic review. J Prosthodont. 2022;31(7):e21. https://doi.org/10.1111/jopr.13464.
6. Sarafidou K, Vasileiadi G, Louvrou MK, Moldovani E, Koidis P, Kokoti M, Bakopoulou A. Screwmentable implant-supported prostheses: a systematic review. J Prosthet Dent. 2022;130(1):35–47. https://doi.org/10.1016/j.prosdent.2021.08.027.
7. Papaspyridakos P, Chen CJ, Chuang SK, Weber HP, Gallucci GO. A systematic review of biologic and technical complications with fixed implant rehabilitations for edentulous patients. Int J Oral Maxillofac Implants. 2012;27:102–10.
8. Thomason JM, Lund JP, Chehade A, Feine JS. Patient satisfaction with mandibular implant overdentures and conventional dentures 6 months after delivery. Int J Prosthodont. 2003;16:467–73. https://doi.org/10.1016/j.prosdent.2003.12.011.

9. Duong H-Y, Roccuzzo A, Stähli A, Salvi GE, Lang NP, Sculean A. Oral health-related quality of life of patients rehabilitated with fixed and removable implant-supported dental prostheses. Periodontol 2000. 2022;88:202–39. https://doi.org/10.1111/prd.12419.
10. Feine JS, Carlsson GE, Awad MA, Chehade A, Duncan WJ, Gizani S, Wismeijer D. The McGill consensus statement on overdentures. Mandibular two-implant overdentures as first choice standard of care for edentulous patients. Gerodontology. 2002;19(1):3–4.
11. Thomason JM, Feine J, Exley C, Moynihan P, Müller F, Naert I, Ellis JS, Barclay C, Butterworth C, Scott B, Lynch C. Mandibular two implant-supported overdentures as the first choice standard of care for edentulous patients-the York consensus statement. Br Dent J. 2009;207(4):185–6.
12. Nedir R, Bischof M, Szmukler-Moncler S, Belser UC, Samson J. Prosthetic complications with dental implants: from an up-to-8-year experience in private practice. Int J Oral Maxillofac Implants. 2006;21:919–28. PMID: 17190302.
13. Payne AGT, Alsabeeha NHM, Atieh MA, Esposito M, Ma S, Anas E-WM. Interventions for replacing missing teeth: attachment systems for implant overdentures in edentulous jaws. Cochrane Database Syst Rev. 2018;10:CD008001. https://doi.org/10.1002/14651858.CD008001.pub2.

# 7 Clinical Applications of Digital Workflow in Dental Implantology

Cemal Ucer

This chapter will look at the application of 3D technology and digital workflow (DWF) in the provision of implant dentistry. Various components of the DWF will be discussed, including intraoral scanning, cone beam computed tomography (CBCT), computer-aided-design/computer-aided-manufacturing (CAD/CAM) processes, milling, additive manufacturing and 3D printing, guided implant surgery, custom-made bone regeneration technique and custom-made implants.

Table 7.1 lists some of the common applications of digital dentistry (DD) in dental implantology.

**Table 7.1** Applications of digital dentistry in dental implantology

| |
|---|
| Assessment and treatment planning—CBCT, IOS, DSD |
| CBCT-based surgical guide design and 3D printing |
| Three-dimensional guided surgery and immediate loading |
| Temporary restoration design (CAD) and 3D printing and milling |
| Intraoral scanning |
| Laboratory scanning |
| CAD/CAM |
| CEREC chairside scanning and CAD/CAM milling |

C. Ucer (✉)
ICE Postgraduate Dental Institute and Hospital, University of Salford, Salford, UK
e-mail: ucer@icedental.institute



C. Barclay (ed.), *Oral Implantology: Assessment to Maintenance*, BDJ Clinician's Guides, https://doi.org/10.1007/978-3-031-55241-0_7

## 7.1 Introduction

Digital dentistry (DD) is a fast-developing, innovative field of dentistry that involves the use of digital technologies and devices that incorporate computer-assisted components to carry out dental procedures instead of using mechanical processes. Following rapid advances made in this field during the last decade, DD is increasingly being used to perform traditional dental procedures more efficiently than using mechanical tools, for restorative, surgical, orthodontic as well as diagnostic imaging purposes. Digital techniques aim to streamline the delivery of dental treatments and help to meet rising patient expectations. Whilst it could easily be seen as a gimmick, emerging research and clinical evidence demonstrate many real benefits of using digital workflow (DWF) in different branches of dentistry. The objective of this chapter is to look at the role of DWF and summarise the fast-developing applications of this technology with special reference to dental implantology.

## 7.2 The Digital Workflow and Computer-Aided Design and Manufacture (CAD/CAM) Technology in Dentistry

CAD/CAM technique involves three distinct stages:

(a) Data acquisition that captures 3D data from an area of interest. In dental implantology, this data includes CBCT diagnostic imaging of the supporting hard tissues and intraoral optical scanning (IOS) of the surface anatomy of the dental structures and soft tissues.
(b) Computer-aided design (CAD) that involves using DWF software (e.g. 3Shape, Exocad, in Lab (Dentsply/Sirona) for creation of virtual models which permit the production of 3D objects or models such as surgical drill guides or dental restorations.
(c) Computer-assisted manufacturing (CAM) which utilises devices such as 3D stereolithographic, LCD or DLP printers or 3D milling units (e.g. CEREC/Primescan milling unit). Final products can be manufactured using a variety of materials such as hybrid ceramic-reinforced composites, metal, zirconium oxide, polymethyl methacrylate (PMMA) or Polyetheretherketone (PEEK) through 3D printing, metal sintering or milling processes.

**Digital Intraoral Cameras (IOCs)** are optical cameras used commonly to produce intraoral images of the mouth. These can be great educational aids and help in the diagnosis and planning stages of treatment as well as in the documentation of cases. IOCs with optical scanning features can also be used for taking "digital impressions". Some IOCs can be used for shade-matching, which could be a valuable adjunct to the traditional shade-matching technique.

**Intraoral Optical Scanning (IOS) Devices:** Intraoral optical scanning (IOS) has been used in restorative dentistry as part of CAD/CAM process for more than a couple of decades (e.g. CEREC/Dentsply). Although the repeatability and precision of IOS are under constant development, dental restorations fabricated with IOS have already been shown to have clinical accuracy that is comparable to conventional techniques with real advantages such as greatly improved workflow efficiency and savings in time and costs. Randomised double-blinded trials demonstrated these advantages, including digitally produced restorations having significantly smaller marginal and internal fit with better interproximal contacts. A review of the literature suggested that digital revolution in restorative dentistry will expand rapidly to become the mainstream mode of restorative design and manufacturing in the next few years.

The CEREC system was introduced by Sirona (Germany) in late 1980s as the first IOS digital impression CAD/CAM device. It has undergone significant developments, including the introduction of Bluecam, Omnicam and, recently, the Primescan versions. The latter no longer requires the use of intraoral opaque powder due to the superior characteristics of its image acquisition camera and can be used to produce single-tooth, quadrant or full-arch 3D images for CAD/CAM processing. After the completion of intraoral scanning, the data can either be processed chair-side for in-house milling (e.g. a single e-max implant crown) or transmitted to a laboratory for the production of crowns, veneers, bridges or surgical guides remotely (Fig. 7.1).

There are several IOS devices already in use in implant dentistry with functionality comparable to that of CEREC technology. These include iTero (uses parallel confocal imaging), which is an open system that can be used to take "digital impressions" for production of crowns, partial or fully removable prostheses, veneers, implants, aligners and retainers using a variety of milling units. It exports digital image files in a Standard Tessellation Language (TSL) format, which can be shared by any other lab equipped with a CAD/CAM system. Although CEREC is a closed system that exports to Sirona's own CAM devices, such as CEREC MCXL, or lab milling units, the latest version—Primescan—can export implant digital impressions in STL format that can also be used by other CAM software (e.g. Exocad, 3Shape) or milling devices. Another market-leading IOS system—3Shape

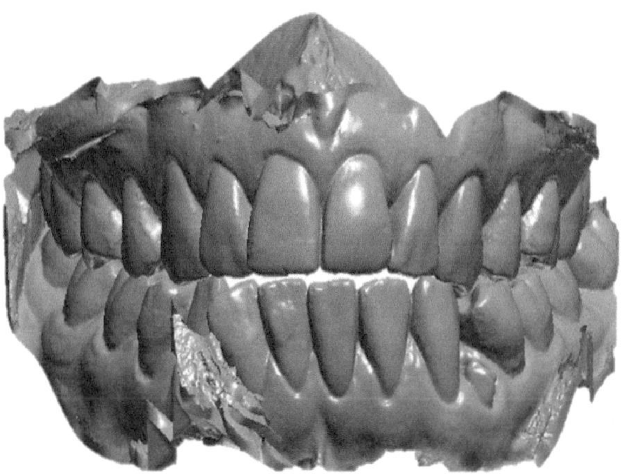

**Fig. 7.1** An STL file acquired from an intraoral scan

(TRIOS)—uses ultrafast optical sectioning and confocal microscopy and can be used to scan for digital manufacturing of partial or full dentures.

Most IOS devices use plastic or metal scan bodies, which are like digital impression posts and are attached to the implant during the scanning process (fixture-level scanning).

## 7.3 Clinical Advantages of DWF

The digital fabrication of dental restorations or drill guides is fast becoming a standard procedure in dental implantology. Using DWF, single- or multiple-unit implant restorations can be constructed without a physical model, thus reducing the time from implant placement to final delivery to a minimum of two or three appointments (Fig. 7.2). Alternatively, restorations can be constructed on 3D-printed dental models with simplified laboratory as well as chairside procedures. Lee et al. have demonstrated many benefits of adapting the DWF over conventional restorative techniques.

Using 3D DWF techniques, implants can now be virtually placed, and surgical drill guides and prefabricated restorations can be produced before actual implant placements to allow immediate implant placement with immediate loading.

These benefits include saving on the cost of impression materials, reducing the stages and overall duration of the restorative treatment, thus significantly improving the cost-effectiveness and efficiency of treatment. Furthermore, it has been shown that patients generally prefer digital impressions (IOS) over conventional analogue impressions.

Another significant benefit of DWF in implant dentistry is that it helps to avoid repeated changes of healing and restorative abutments by allowing implant restoration to be constructed with fewer number of restorative stages. The so-called "one-abutment/one-time" technique has been shown to lead to significantly less bone loss at the bone–implant interface by enhancing soft-tissue maturation and stability as a result of reducing repeated soft-tissue trauma to the peri-implant mucosal seal (Fig. 7.3).

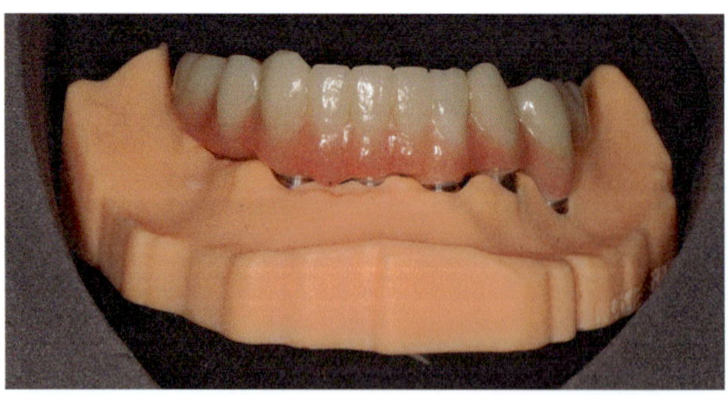

**Fig. 7.2** 3D printed stereolithographic dental model and CAD/CAM-manufactured full-arch mandibular bridge

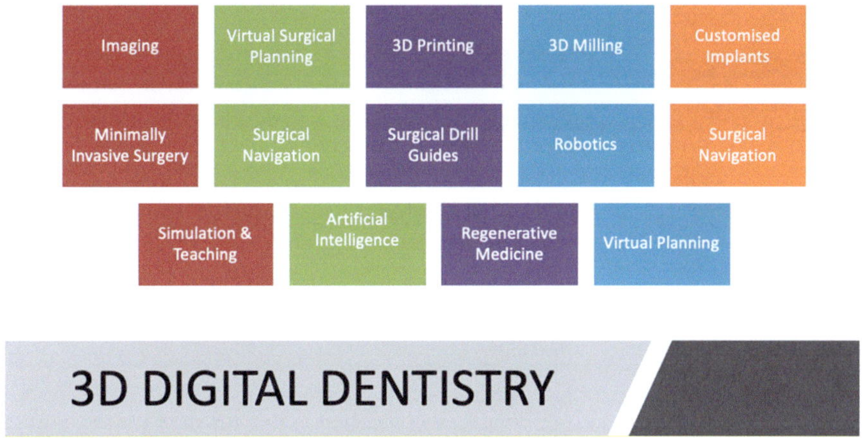


**Fig. 7.3** Applications of 3D digital workflow in implant dentistry: current clinical and experimental data suggests that improved surgical accuracy and precision can be achieved when placing dental implants using guided surgery compared to free-hand drilling techniques. However, the limitations and shortcomings of DWF must be recognised to avoid complications occurring when using the guided surgical techniques. Some of the dental applications of DWF are shown below

## 7.4 Digital Workflow for Surgical Guide Production

A significant contribution of DWF to dental implantology has been the introduction of 3D-printed surgical drill guide technique, which uses both the CBCT images and the intraoral surface images of hard and soft tissues of the mouth. 3D surgical guides help to transfer the virtual implant planning, designed using CBCT software, into prosthodontically and anatomically guided implant positions in the jawbone with surgical accuracy. This undoubtedly offers distinct advantages over acrylic drill guides produced in the laboratory on plaster casts with no reference to cross-sectional-derived radiological information.

The key stages of DWF for the design and production of a surgical guide are outlined in Figs. 7.4 and 7.5. The process begins with the acquisition of the CBCT scan of the region of interest (using the national diagnostic imaging guidelines and justification criteria).

A surface scan of the teeth and the mucosa is taken either with an IOS device or using a conventional analogue impression. The latter is scanned in the laboratory to generate an STL file of the intraoral images. The STL file and the Digital Imaging and Communications in Medicine (DICOM) datasets are then imported into 3D CAD software (e.g., Implant Studio or BlueSkyBio).

Computer-aided surgical guide design allows highly accurate assessment of the available bone quality and quantity at the implant site. This facilitates the prosthodontically and anatomically guided most optimum implant placement surgery. An implant restoration such as a crown, bridge or even a full-arch bridge could be

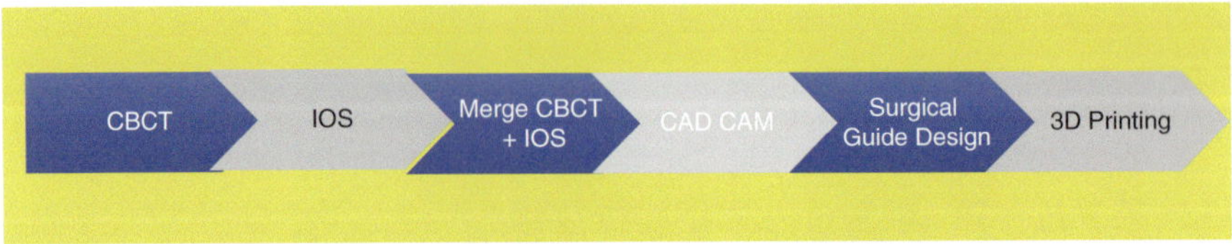


**Fig. 7.4** DWF involves the CBCT and IOS image acquisition stages followed by merging of radiological and optical scan data using a 3D CAD software such as Implant Studio (3Shape) or Co-Diagnostics (Straumann)

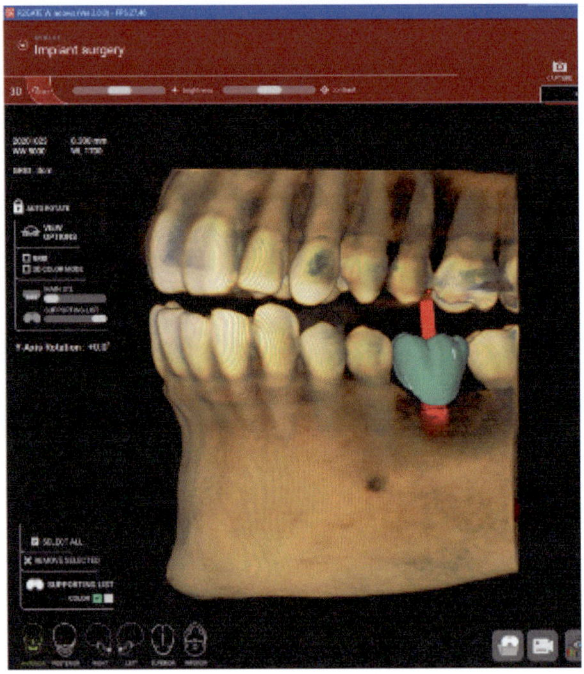


**Fig. 7.5** STL file of IOS and CBCT DICOM images are merged in the CAD software (e.g. BlueSkyBio) for virtual implant placement and surgical guide design. The surgical guide is exported in STL format and sent to a 3D printer for the manufacturing of the surgical guide in resin

wwdesigned and prefabricated to fit on the virtually planned implant for immediavte implant loading.

Virtual implant placement is carried out using the 3D CAD diagnostic and treatment planning software. This allows the fabrication of a fully guided surgical stent designed to optimise implant placement within the alveolar bone. A crown is designed and fabricated either from a dental resin or milled in zirconium for immediate loading. A print-out obtained from the software specifies the selected implant type, diameter, length and the required drill depth (Figure 7.6).

The implant is placed after preparing the implant osteotomy through the surgical guide. In this case, the surgical guide is tooth-supported (Fig. 7.7).

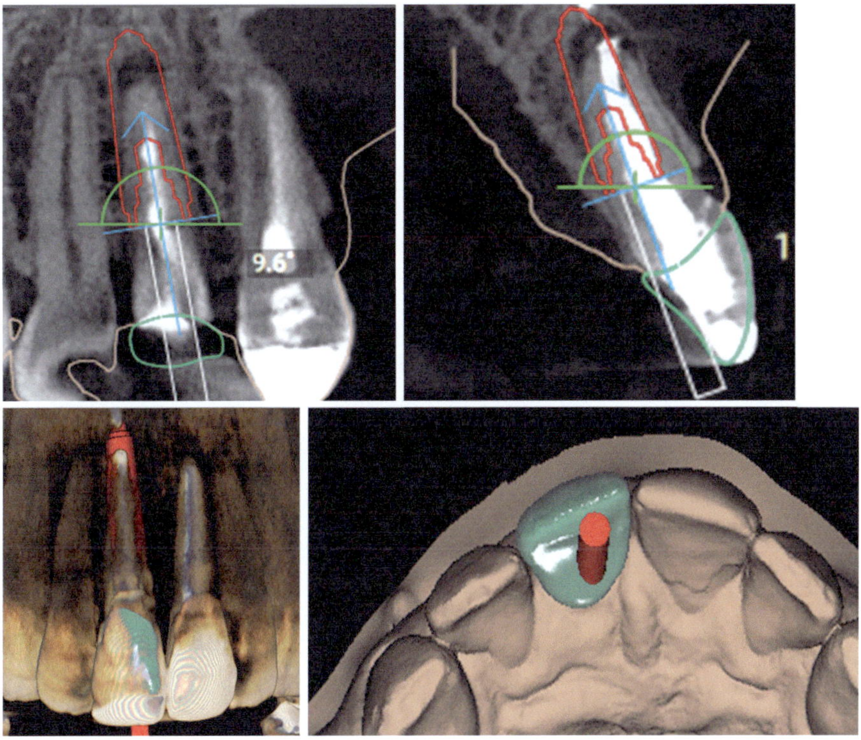


**Fig. 7.6** Guided surgical navigation optimises the 3D implant placement whilst protecting the adjacent vital structures. DWF also helps to improve communication between the clinician, the laboratory and the patient. The images below illustrate the planning stages of 3D virtual implant placement using R2Gate ® software

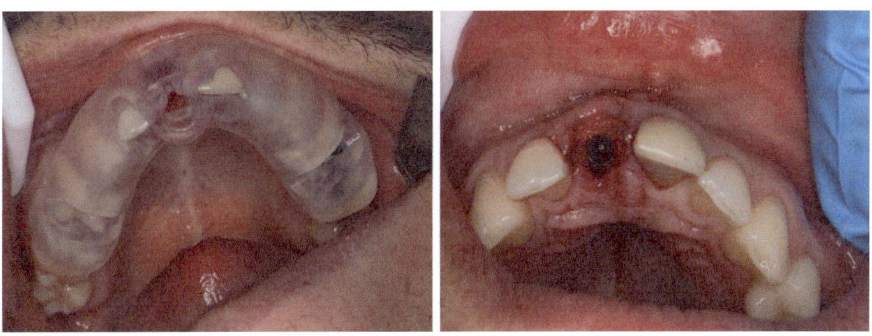

**Fig. 7.7** Tooth-supported 3D printed surgical guide is used for implant placement of a central incisor

The software highlights the quality of the bone at the implant interface. This information can be useful in modifying the surgical protocol and/or implant type selection in order to maximise the primary stability. It can also help to determine the healing period more objectively, especially if the bone type at the interface is found to be the soft-type D4 bone.

Surgical plan and drilling instructions are printed out to be used during implant placement. Implant type, diameter, length, sleeve offset and order number are specified. Drilling instructions specify the drill length that should be drilled with reference to the top of the drill guide cylinder.

## 7.5 3D Printing of Surgical Guide

The STL file of the surgical guide designed within a CAD software programme (e.g. Implant Studio) is imported into a 3D printer (e.g. FormLabs-3, Rapid Shape). After the 3D printing process, the surgical guide requires a systematic postprocessing, which involves cleaning, washing in isopropyl alcohol solution and the final curing steps. These are critical stages which can significantly affect the dimensional stability and accuracy of the guide.

**Table: Types of Surgical Guides:**

(a) Drill guides
(b) Fully guided surgical guides
(c) Bone reduction guides
(d) Stackable surgical guides for immediate loading
(e) Zygomatic implant guides
(f) Maxillary sinus access cavity guides

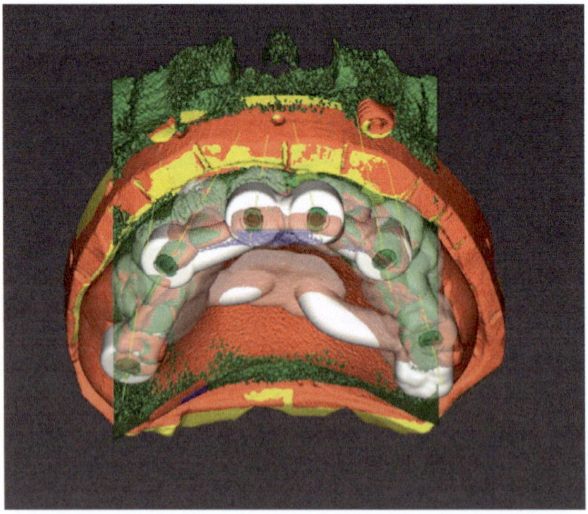

**Fig. 7.8** Static 3D guide design: a mucosa-supported surgical guide

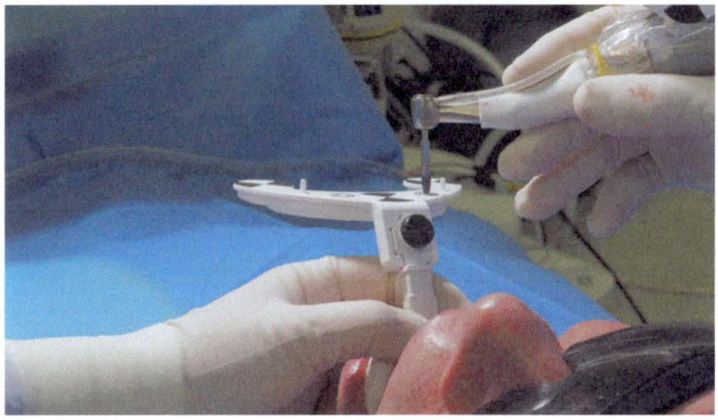

**Fig. 7.9** Dynamic guides such as the Navident allow for CBCT-based real-time navigational surgery

**Table: Classification of Surgical Guides According to Supporting Structures**

(a) Tooth-supported guides
(b) Mucosa-supported guides (Fig. 7.8)
(c) Bone-supported guides
(d) Screw marker-supported guides

**Table: Types of Surgical Placement**

(a) Static
(b) Dynamic

Surgical guides can be milled, sintered in Co-Cr or 3D printed using dental resin.

Computer-aided dynamic navigation system is designed to virtually plan implant restorations and execute, in real-time, dental implant placement surgery (Fig. 7.9). The patient's CBCT scan is linked with fiduciary markers attached to the teeth or the jaw bone. The patient, CBCT dataset and the hand-piece are then linked optically to allow the surgeon to place the implant whilst monitoring the drill or the implant advancing in real time on the screen with reference to adjacent structures, nerves and the preplanned implant site. Dynamic navigation offers certain advantages over static guided surgery, such as avoiding the need for 3D manufacturing of stereolithographic guides. It also makes it possible to make changes to the implant plan (e.g. number of implants, length, diameter and implant position) intraoperatively.

## 7.6 3D Fully Guided Surgery and Immediate Loading

Fully guided implant placement: Implant is placed through the surgical guide immediately after implant bed preparation. Three-dimensional assessment, planning and prosthodontically and anatomically guided (PAG) surgery using drill guides can improve the surgical accuracy and avoid surgical complications. DWF also improves the restorative accuracy of implant placement in ideal bony sites under optimum loading conditions (Figs. 7.10, 7.11, 7.12, and 7.13).

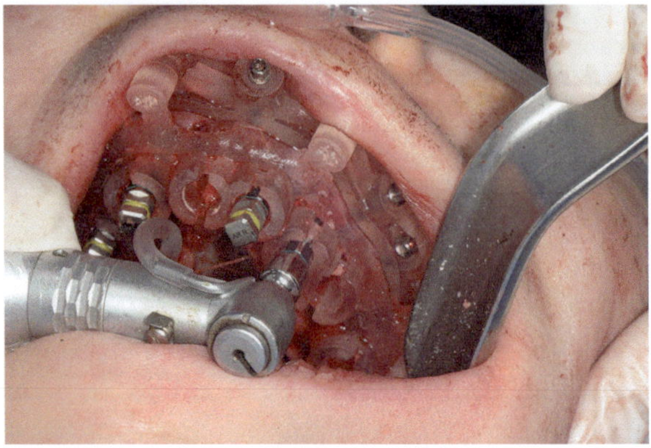

**Fig. 7.10** Clinical applications of DWF—Full arch implant rehabilitation of a fully edentulous maxilla with irregular residual alveolar ridge. Computer guided implant placement technique streamlines the treatment whilst improving the surgical accuracy and precision

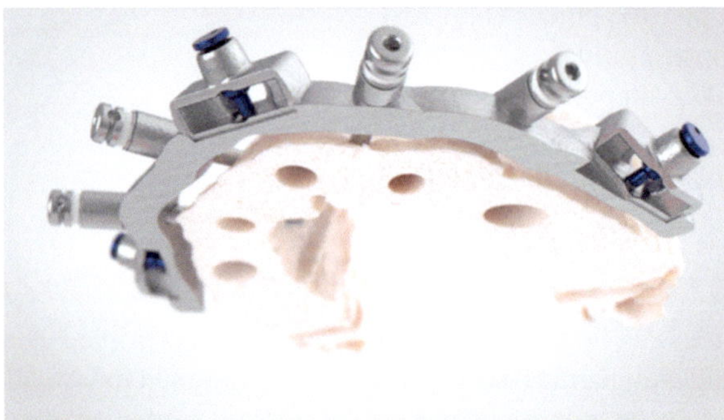

**Fig. 7.11** 3D printed bone reduction guide is designed to prepare the alveolar ridge for implant placement when the alveolar ridge is irregular or uneven. This image shows part of a stackable surgical guide system (Chrome®) 3D printed in metal for increased rigidity and accuracy (CHROME®, Quoris 3D, Courtesy of Dr James Hamill)

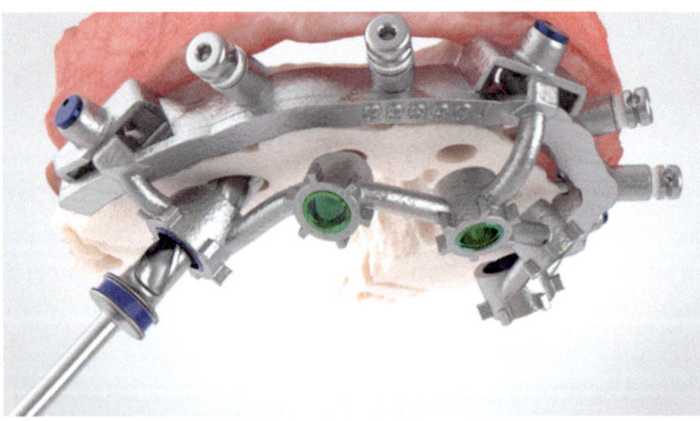

**Fig. 7.12** A fully guided surgical protocol allows the use of a series of pin-supported stack-up guides for preplanned bone reduction followed by guided implant bed preparation. After implant placement, a 3D printed interim prosthesis is connected to the implant abutments for immediate loading. (CHROME®, Quoris 3D, Courtesy of Dr James Hamill)

CHROME® is an example of a highly structured, fully guided implant placement and immediate loading technique that involves using a stackable devices of 3D printed metal drill guides and loading templates.

After preparing the irregular alveolar ridge using a bone reduction guide, implant placement guide is connected to the base plate for implant bed preparation followed by preplanned, fully guided implant insertion

Implants are placed using a fully guided implant placement template attached to the CHROME® frame, which is anchored to the ridge by means of horizontal bone pins or screws (Figs. 7.14 and 7.15).

Next, temporary cylinders are connected to the multi-unit abutments (MUA), and an interim full-arch bridge is connected to the prosthetic cylinders chairside.

The interim prosthesis is connected to the temporary cylinders, and abutment screw holes are covered with a temporary filling material (Figs. 7.14, 7.15, and 7.16).

Fully guided surgery allows the placement of dental implants and immediate loading; the final prosthesis is prefabricated using CAD/CAM, and a fully guided surgical drill guide is used to position the implants before connecting the bridgework immediately.

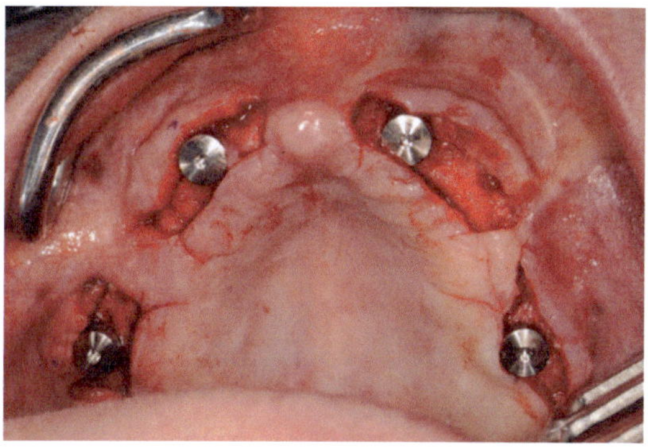

**Fig. 7.13** A fully guided technique allows minimally invasive implant placement. After implant placement, multi-unit abutments are connected to the implants

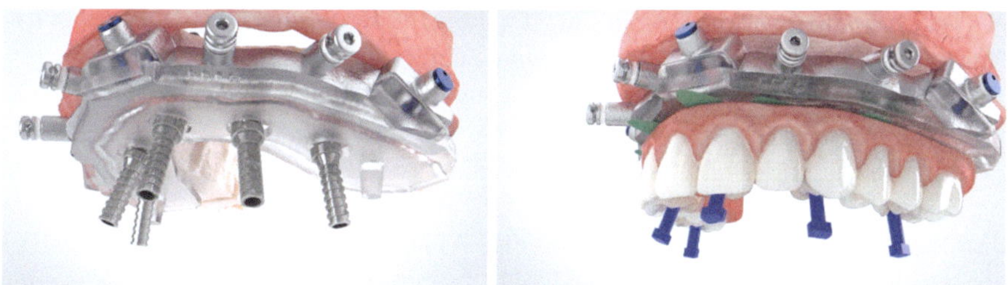

**Fig. 7.14** Temporary cylinders are connected to the MUA using a stackable guides system. These images show how Chrome® system which uses stackable guides, facilitate the placement of implants followed by connection of an interim restaoration for immediate full arch loading (CHROME®, Quoris 3D, Courtesy of Dr James Hamill)

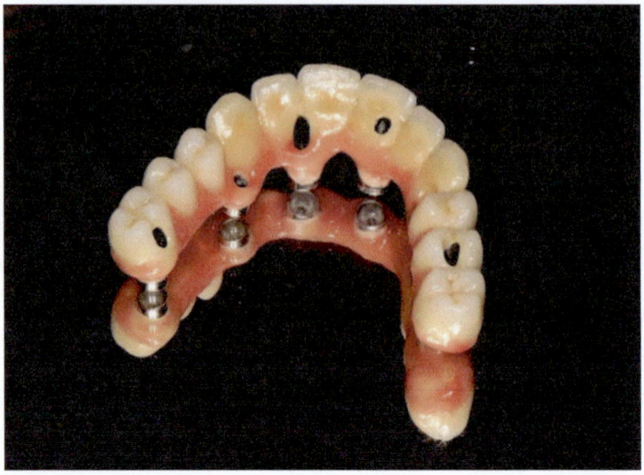

**Fig. 7.15** A 3D planned, restorative and surgically guided full-arch bridge ready to be fitted

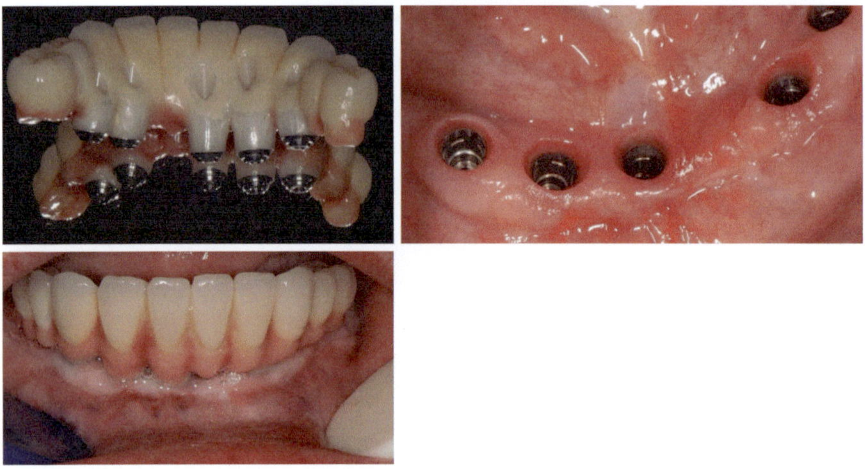

**Fig. 7.16** Images below illustrate fitting of a full arch mandibular bridgework after placement of implants using guided surgery

This type of surgical guide allows for preparation of implant osteotomies followed by immediate placement of implants and immediate loading of implant restorations such as all-on-4 or all-on-6 bridgework.

Other applications of 3D surgical guides:

3D surgical guides have been used for

(a) Placement of zygomatic implants (Fig. 7.17)
(b) Drill guides for harvesting bone blocks from the mandible when reconstructing intraoral bone defects
(c) Drill guides for removal of the lateral wall of the maxillary sinus when performing lateral wall sinus grafting

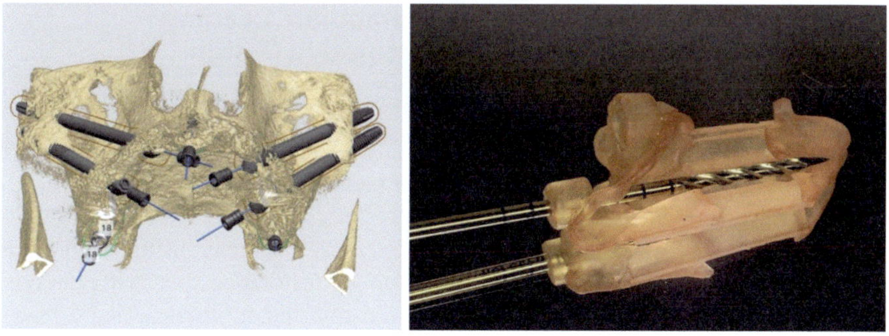

**Fig. 7.17** Computer planning and a 3D surgical guide used for placement of a zygomatic implant

(d) Placement of implants using the crestal sinus lift technique
(e) Gingival lengthening
(f) Endodontics
(g) OVD registration during digital intraoral scanning

The planning and placement of zygomatic implants benefit from 3D planning, as these fixtures are placed in close proximity of highly vascular vital structures such as the orbit, infraorbital nerve and the infratemporal fossa. In complex cases, surgical planning usually involves a trial run using prefabricated 3D stereolithographic models of the maxilla before the actual implants are placed.

## 7.7 Clinical Applications: 3D Prosthodontically and Anatomically Guided Immediate Implant Placement with Immediate Loading

Using 3D DWF, a dental implant can be placed within a fresh extraction site immediately at the time of tooth removal and immediately loaded with a CAD/CAM restoration. There are two techniques available for this procedure in suitable patients:

(a) Prefabricated crown designed using CAD/CAM software as part of guided surgical DWF. The tooth to be extracted is virtually removed from the DICOM images of the jaw (virtual extraction technique). A dental implant is then inserted into the scan using a virtual implant design tool. A 3D surgical guide is planned and printed to allow the placement of the implant following tooth removal. Subject to achieving good primary stability, the prefabricated milled crown is attached to the implant using a Ti-base abutment.
(b) CEREC chairside workflow: Following extraction and Immediate implant placement CEREC workflow is used to design and mill a crown for immediate loading.

## 7.8 Immediate Placement and Immediate Loading with Chairside CAD/CAM Restorative Design and Manufacture

Abutment (ti-base) with a milled crown is connected to the implant for immediate loading. Final restoration is provided 3 months later when hard and soft tissue maturation has been completed (Fig. 7.18)

Chairside computer-aided implant restoration design and manufacture technique:

A prescription is filled in for the desired implant restoration specifying the type of the implant system, desired abutment type (customised or prefabricated ti-base), materials to be used (e.g. emax, ZirOxide, titanium)

After intraoral scanning using a dedicated implant scanbody, the acquired STL file is imported into the CAD software, and the scanbody is aligned accurately with a scanbody image of the implant system from the CAD library (Fig. 7.19).

CAD software (e.g. 3 Shape or Exocad) calculates and proposes a restoration using anatomical and biomimetic algorithms. This proposed restoration is then modified using various tools available in the tool menu. A virtual articulator is also available. For single crowns, this process can be completed virtually without using a physical model (3Shape chairside or CEREC) (Fig. 7.20).

Emergence profile is customised to fit the soft tissue margin optimally. Note the colour coding used to ensure that the customised abutment is not over- or under-built with reference to the marginal tissue contour.

Once the final crown and the abutment have been designed using CAD software, the prosthesis is exported in an STL format. The separate files for the abutment and the crown are sent to a three- or five-axis milling machine or to a laboratory for manufacturing using a CAM software (Fig. 7.21).

A CEREC machine (e.g. Primemill) can manufacture an implant crown designed using a chairside CAD/CAM software (CEREC®) in as little as 8–10 min for immediate fitting.

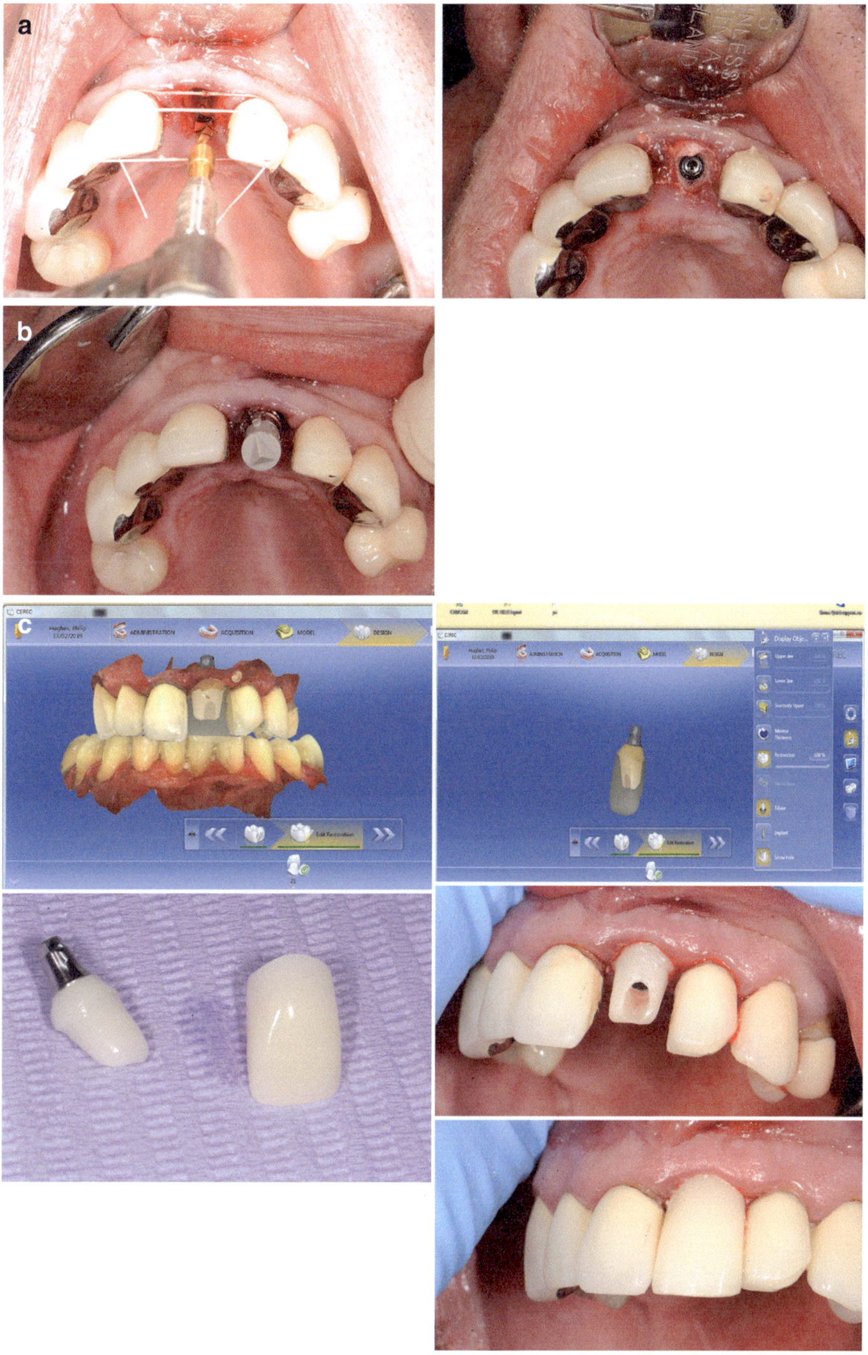


**Fig. 7.18** (**a**) After a minimally traumatic extraction using a periotome and/or piezo surgery, an implant is placed into the fresh extraction site. The peri-implant gap is filled with a graft such as xenograft or alloplast. (**b**) CEREC scanbody is attached to the implant and IOS is carried out. (**c**) An abutment and a crown are designed using CEREC chairside software

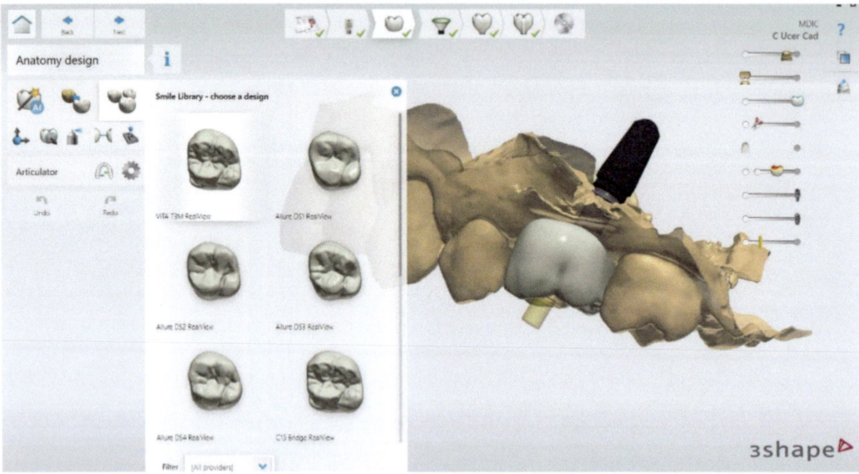


**Fig. 7.19** Digital plan

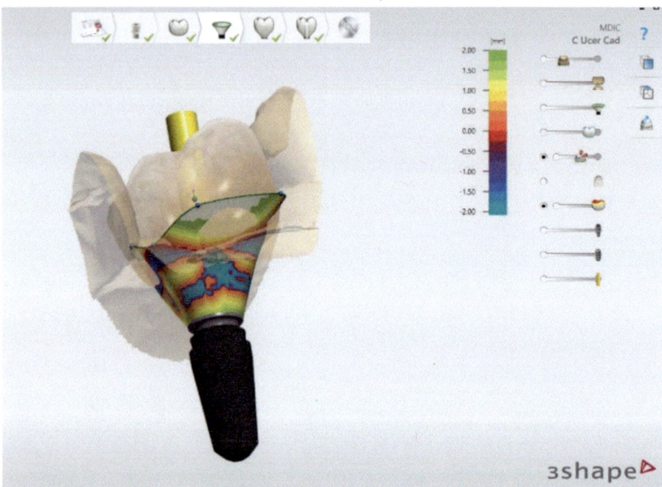


**Fig. 7.20** Proposed restoration

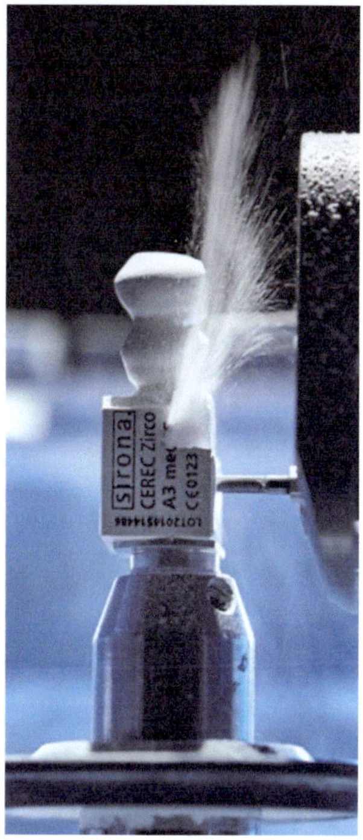


**Fig. 7.21** Milling

## 7.9 Other Clinical Applications of DWF: Bioprinting

Bioprinting is a method used to fabricate scaffolds for tissue engineering. Additive manufacturing (AM) techniques, such as fused deposition modelling (FDM) or stereolithography (SLA), and substractive manufacturing techniques, such as milling, are being used increasingly in recent years to produce biomaterials for tissue regeneration, including blood vessels, urethra, trachea, bone and soft tissues. Metal powder (e.g. titanium or cobalt-chrome) and synthetic polymers, such as polylactic acid (PLA), polyglycolic acid (PGA), polylactic-glycolic acid (PLGA), PMMA and PEEK, have been used to produce implantable biomaterials.

In implant dentistry, 3D DWF has been used to produce novel devices such as customised bone grafts (e.g. Puros CAD/CAM allograft block by Zimvie), bone graft plates and meshes (e.g. accuramesh by Zimvie) as well as individualised 3D printed titanium subperiosteal full-arch implants in order to overcome the complexity and morbidity of major bone graft surgery that is often required for the rehabilitation of patients who present with severe bone atrophy or oncology bone defects.

## 7.10 3D CAD/CAM Customised Allograft for Reconstruction of Vertical Intraoral Bone Defects

This technique involves CAD/CAM production of block bone grafts or plates made of allografts for reconstruction of large vertical and horizontal alveolar bone defects. A preoperative CBCT scan of the area of interest is used to design and mill a bone graft of customised dimensions both vertically and horizontally. This technique is indicated for the reconstruction of large intraoral defects as an alternative to more invasive and complex autogenic bone harvesting and defect reconstruction surgery (Fig. 7.22).

Bone graft is designed using DWF and produced using allograft bone material. The prescribed implant length and diameter are used to determine the amount of bone grafting necessary to accommodate the selected implants. The bone graft is secured in place using small bone screws via a simple soft-tissue access surgery (Figs. 7.23, 7.24, and 7.25).

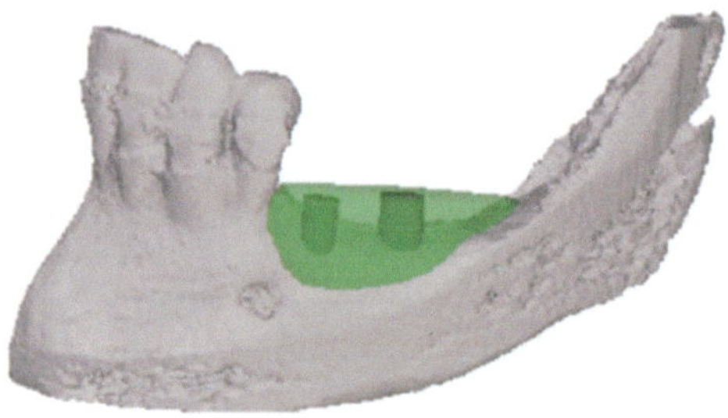

**Fig. 7.22** 3D computer aided bone graft planning

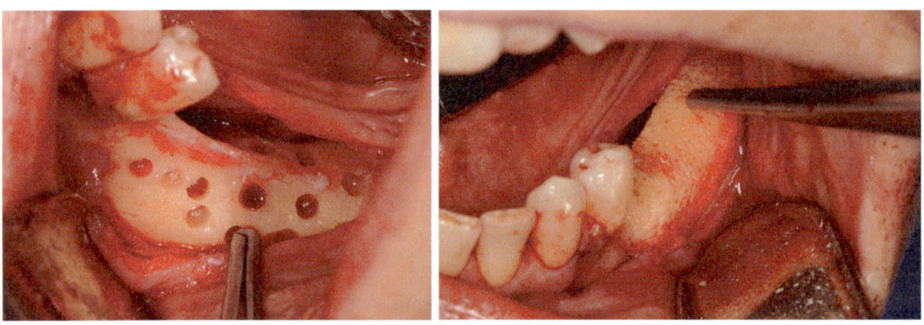

**Fig. 7.23** Occlusal view of the allograft (ZimVie®) in situ

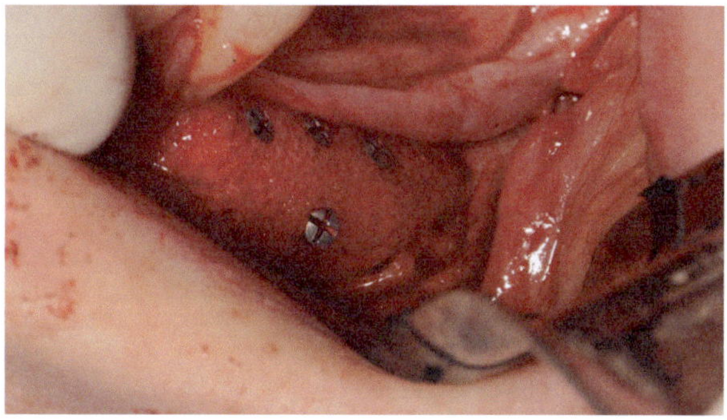

**Fig. 7.24** A patient-specific CAD/CAM-produced bone graft is inserted subperiosteally and secured to the residual ridge using bone screws

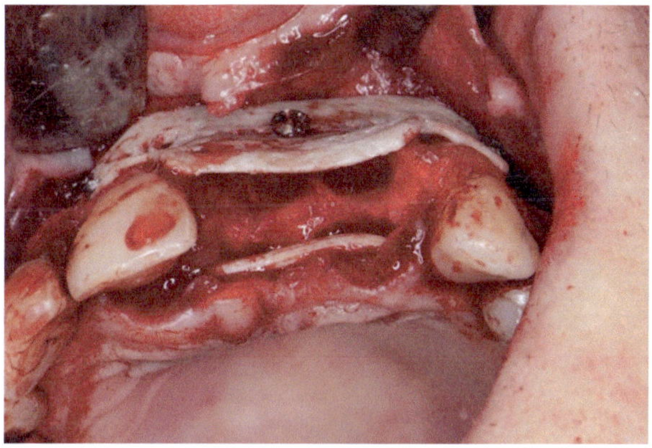

**Fig. 7.25** An alternative to the titanium mesh technique is the use of CAD/CAM manufactured customised bone plates (ZimVie Biomaterials), which is particularly indicated in the regeneration of bone in vertical and horizontal planes

## 7.11 3D CAD/CAM-Customised Titanium Mesh for the Construction of Horizontal and Vertical Bone Defects

Gross atrophy of the alveolar bone in the posterior mandible presents several challenges for dental rehabilitation of the patient. Autogenic bone grafting requires a second surgical site either intra- or extraorally and is prone to complications with significant risk of morbidity. Techniques such as GBR are therefore employed to reduce the complexity of grafting procedures. Custom-produced titanium mesh is a form of guided bone regeneration, which reduces the complexity of surgery even further (Fig. 7.26).

The amount of required bone regeneration is calculated with reference to the available bone volume of the defect and the desired dimensions of the implants to be placed. A customised titanium mesh is then manufactured to fit over the defect to allow vertical and horizontal bone regeneration (Fig. 7.27).

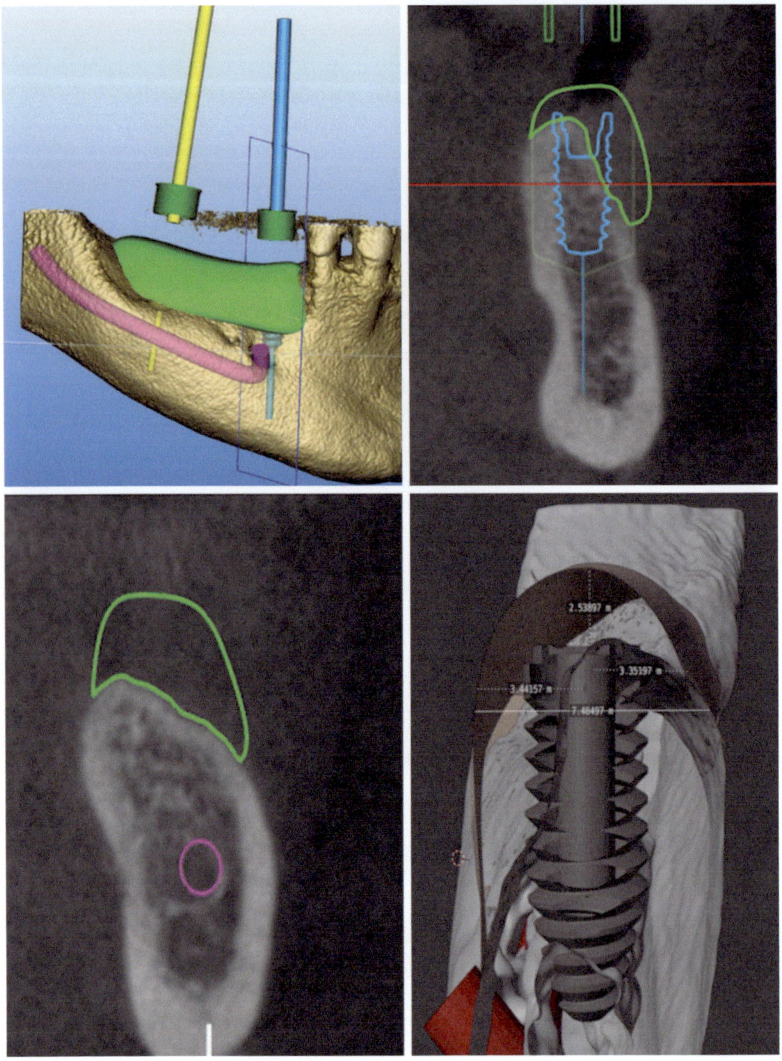

**Fig. 7.26** A 3D planning software (e.g. Real Guide®) is used to design a titanium mesh (e.g AccuraMesh®) customised to achieve the optimum bone regeneration to support the implant. Green lines show the amount of vertical bone required to support the implant

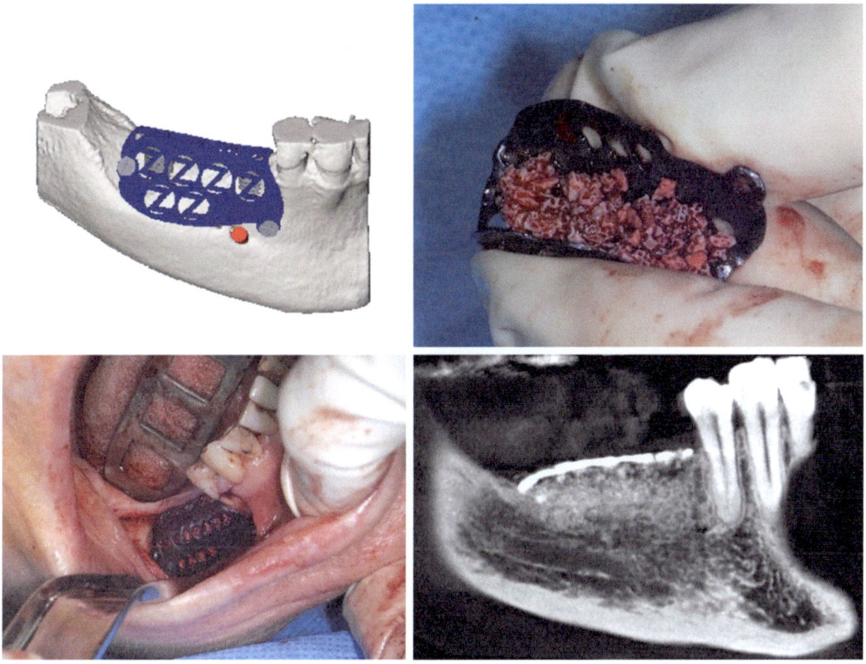

**Fig. 7.27** A custom titanium mesh produced from a CBCT image (Accuramesh®, ZimVie), filled with a mixture of autogenic graft and a xenograft, is placed in the posterior mandible for regeneration of large horizontal and vertical bone defect. A postoperative CBCT data showing significant amount of vertical and horizontal bone regeneration that has taken place in 4 months within the defect covered by the titanium mesh

## 7.12 Patient-Specific Additively Manufactured Titanium Subperiosteal Dental Implants

There are limited options available for oral implant rehabilitation in patients suffering from severe alveolar atrophy. The gold standard has been autogenic bone grafting with bone harvested from the mandible or extraorally. This undoubtedly increases the complexity of the treatment. Extraoral bone grafting is resource-demanding and involves more serious risk of complications and morbidity. Alternatives include maxillary sinus grafting when possible, use of tilted implants, short implants, zygomatic and pterygoid implants with relative advantages and disadvantages. Subperiosteal implants were introduced a few decades ago for the rehabilitation of patients with severe atrophy as an alternative to major autogenic bone grafting. The clinical use of subperiosteal implants was largely abandoned over time with the success of endosseous titanium implants.

With the emergence of digital technology and the application of additive manufacturing processes, patient-specific 3D printed subperiosteal implants have been re-gaining popularity in implant dentistry.

An innovative additively manufactured subperiosteal jaw implant (AMSJI) concept (CADskills BV, Ghent, Belgium) was introduced recently. The AMSJI consists of two subunits (left and right), which are customised to the maxillary bone anatomy of each patient, based on a CBCT data set. The subunits consist of two wings and a basal looped frame connecting the arms and the transmucosal posts. The wings are situated on the canine and zygomatic buttresses and are fixed in these locations using osteosynthesis screws. Both subunits are connected intraorally by a temporary connector, and the latter by a definitive primary matrix structure.

A recent paper reported on the successful one-year review of these implants with minimal adverse bone remodelling. If the results are confirmed in long-term studies, this relatively straightforward technique that could be carried out under a local anaesthetic will offer significant advantages over more invasive techniques that are indicated for the rehabilitation of a severely atrophic jaw (Fig. 7.28).

The two subunits of the AMSJI subperiosteal implant connected intraorally. The implants are fixed to the maxillary and zygomatic bones at strategic points of the dense cortical bone using osseosynthesis screws. The two subunits are fitted with a titanium bar that incorporates conventional implant abutments for connection of a fixed full-arch prosthesis (Fig. 7.29).

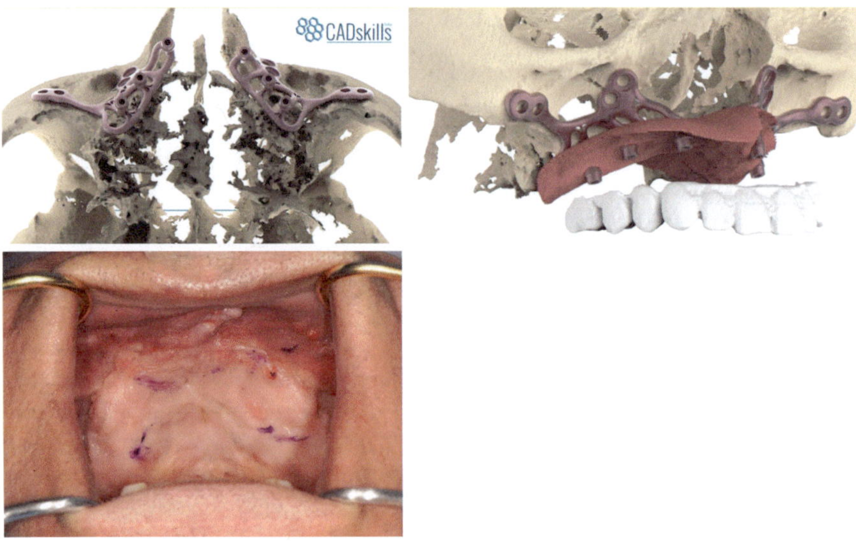


**Fig. 7.28** Reconstruction of severely atrophic maxilla with the AMSJI custom-manufactured subperiosteal implant

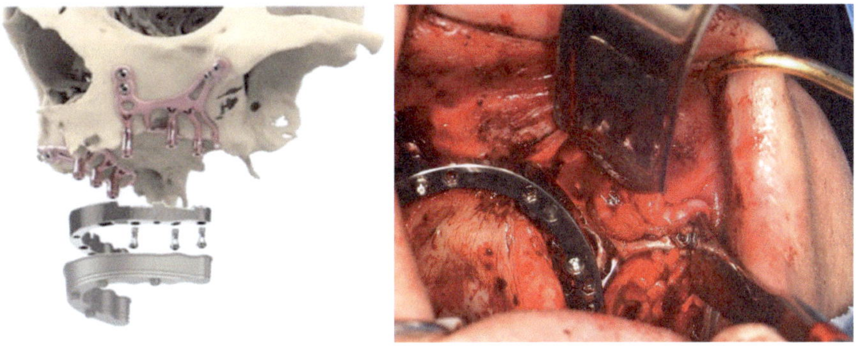

**Fig. 7.29** The two subunits of the AMSJI subperiosteal implant connected intraorally

## 7.13 Accuracy and Limitations of DWF

Trueness is defined as the closeness of a measured value to a standard or a known value. On the other hand, precision refers to the closeness of two or more measurements to each other. Trueness and precision constitute accuracy. Both criteria have been studied in recent years. Research has so far shown that the accuracy of full-arch IOS and model-free restorations is clinically acceptable and compatible with that obtained from conventional analogue impressions. Surgical guide design, production and clinical efficiency were also shown to be equally good. When an implant is placed using either a guided surgery or a free hand technique, there is always a deviation in all three axes between the planned and actual positions—deviation at entry point (x), deviation at apex (y), angle deviation (z) and error in implant shoulder height.

In a systematic review, a mean accuracy of 1.2 mm at the implant entry point was demonstrated by Thahib. However, there was a large variation between the minimum and maximum values (as much as 7 mm). The authors recommended that a 2-mm clearance during virtual implant placement be given between implants and vital neighbouring structures.

In an randomised clinical trial (RCT), Tallarico et al. [1] found that there were differences in accuracy between different surgical guide designs. Amit et al. have concluded that guided surgery, compared to free-hand surgery, improved the margin of error by increasing the surgical accuracy using a novel R2 gate system.

## 7.14 Conclusions

Modern oral implantology and implant prosthodontics depend on comprehensive diagnostics and precise planning to achieve successful outcomes and meet high patient expectations. Prosthodontically and anatomically guided (PAG) 3D surgical implant placement technique offers excellent advantages in achieving functionally, aesthetically and biologically satisfactory results in a highly controlled, predictable and systematic approach.

Recent advances being made in digital dentistry and digital workflow are revolutionising the provision of restorative dentistry as well as dental implantology. DWF is no longer a gimmick but an essential and integral part of the provision of successful modern dental implant treatment. This applies to the replacement of a single tooth as well as the reconstruction of complex hard- and soft-tissue defects and reconstruction of severely atrophic jaws using customised implants and zygomatic implant fixtures. In the field of maxillofacial oncology, reconstruction of large maxillofacial ablation defects using 3D virtual DWF for harvesting of fibular grafts with immediate implant placements and immediate loading using guided surgical techniques has been revolutionising the immediate rehabilitation of patients with severe head and neck defects.

The ability to carry out accurate diagnostic imaging, 3D assessment and treatment planning and accurate execution of the planned treatment using prosthodontically and anatomically guided (PAG) surgical concept has made a significant impact in this field. In fact, the CAD/CAM-supported PAG technique, combined with the design and manufacture of abutments and implant-supported restorations through use of DWF, has created a new standard in implant dentistry that offers almost unlimited design options for the optimum placement of implants with ideal emergence profile, the dimension and angulation of the restorations and dental aesthetics. In addition to financial benefits, it represents a biologically advantageous, one-abutment/one-time approach with customised screw-retained, full-contour crowns or cemented crowns on custom abutments [2]

It must be recognised that the DWF technology is constantly evolving, and guided implant surgery carries its own specific limitations and risks in terms of CAD/CAM manufacturing inaccuracies and application errors. These possible sources of error must be recognised and carefully managed and mitigated to avoid adverse consequences. Although the PAG 3D surgical technique facilitates the accurate positioning of dental implants compared to the free-hand model, currently, the use of this technology is, by no means, mandatory but it certainly helps to improve the quality of treatment by offering better case analysis, planning and execution both surgically and prosthodontically.

One major disadvantage of this digital workflow is the learning curve it requires on behalf of the clinician. Final implant placement will always differ from the planned position, and extreme caution is required when carrying out the surgery. Blind reliance on guided surgical technology would be irresponsible and dangerous. Clinicians undertaking these procedures should be conscious of the fact that good surgical experience and skills are essential to avoid the occurrence of unfortunate complications.

Accuracy-guided surgery depends on several factors, and the errors could be cumulative. Clinicians should, therefore, be experienced in free-hand technique to manage any inaccuracies that they will encounter when using the technology.

In conclusion, the current evidence suggests that prosthodontically and anatomically guided (PAG) DWF workflow provides a safe, smooth and effective treatment alternative to the conventional workflow with many advantages, such as improved safety and efficiency features.

Furthermore, digital workflow allows for better surgical and prosthodontic decision-making, and simplifies the treatment protocols to facilitate better communication with the dental team and the patient. Further developments in this field include the introduction of robotic surgical techniques to dental implantology.

## References


1. Tallarico M, Meloni SM, Canullo L, Caneva M, Polizzi G. Five year esults of a randomised controlled trial comparing patient rehabilitated with immediately loaded maxillary cross-arch fixed dental prosthesis by four or six implants using guided surgery. Clin Implant Dent Relat Res. 2016;18(5):965–72.
2. Beuer F, Groesser J, Schweiger J, Hey J, Güth J-F, Stimmelmayr M. The digital one-abutment/one-time concept. A clinical report. J Prosthodontics. 2015;24(7):580–5.


## Further Reading


Ahrberg D, Lauer HC, Ahrberg M, Weigl P. Evaluation of fit and efficiency of CAD/CAM fabricated all-ceramic restorations based on direct and indirect digitalization: a double-blinded, randomized clinical trial. Clin Oral Investig. 2016;20(2):291–300. https://doi.org/10.1007/s00784-015-1504-6. PMID 26070435.

Lee SJ, Gallucci GO. Digital vs conventional implant impressions: efficiency outcomes. Clin Oral Implants Res. 2013;24:111–5.

Logozzo S, Franceschini G, Kilpela A, et al. A comparative analysis of intraoral 3D digital scanners for restorative dentistry. Int J Med Tech. 2011;5. http://ispub.com/IJMT/5/1/10082

Michelinakis G, Nikolidakis D. Using the surgical guide for impression-free digital bite registration in the edentulous maxilla-a technical note. Int J Implant Dent. 2019;5(1):19. https://doi.org/10.1186/s40729-019-0172-8. PMID: 31115829; PMCID: PMC6529490.

Salah M, Tayebi L, Moharamzadeh K, Naini FB. Three-dimensional bio-printing and bone tissue engineering: technical innovations and potential applications in maxillofacial reconstructive surgery. Maxillofac Plastic Reconstruct Surg. 2020;42:18. https://doi.org/10.1186/s40902-020-00263-6.

Syrek A, Reich G, Ranftl D, Klein C, Cerny B, Brodesser J. Clinical evaluation of all-ceramic crowns fabricated from intraoral digital impressions based on the principle of active wavefront sampling. J Dent. 2010;38(7):553–9. https://doi.org/10.1016/j.jdent.2010.03.015. PMID 20381576.

Tahmaseb A, Wu V, Wismeijer D, Coucke W, Evans C. The accuracy of static computer-aided implant surgery: a systematic review and meta-analysis. Clin Oral Implants Res. 2018;29(Suppl 16):416–35. https://doi.org/10.1111/clr.13346. PMID: 30328191.

Ting-Shu S, Jian S. Intraoral digital impression technique: a review. J Prosthodont. 2015;24:313–21.

Tyndall DA, et al. Position statement of the American Academy of Oral and maxillofacial radiology on selection criteria for the use of radiology in dental implantology with emphasis on cone beam computed tomography. Oral Surg Oral Med Oral Pathol Oral Radiol. 2012;113(6):817–26. https://doi.org/10.1016/j.oooo.2012.03.005.

Van den Borre C, Rinaldi M, De Neef B, Loomans NAJ, Nout E, Van Doorne L, Naert I, Politis C, Schouten H, Klomp G, Beckers L, Freilich MM, Mommaerts MY. Radiographic evaluation of bone remodeling after additively manufactured subperiosteal jaw implantation (AMSJI) in the maxilla: a one-year follow-up study. J Clin Med. 2021;10(16):3542. https://doi.org/10.3390/jcm10163542.

# 8 Occlusion in Implant Dentistry

Stephen Davies, Pete Young, and Amin Aminian

## 8.1 Introduction

The fundamental features of implant treatment for the replacement of missing teeth have not changed since its introduction into mainstream clinical practice in the United Kingdom in the 1980s and, before that, since their conception by Professor Brånemark in 1965 [1, 2],. A comprehensive planning stage is needed before the surgical placement of the implant(s) into sufficient height and width of bone, where an element of stability is required. After a varying time period ranging from immediate loading to a delayed approach, implants are eventually restored with a fixed or removable prosthesis.

The advent of cone beam computed tomography (CBCT) technology was a "gamechanger" in the planning phase while the surgical and restorative stages have also evolved significantly over the years, leading to the digital era. These have included changes in implant design, connection type and material choices. However, the fundamental features of conventional treatment remain unchanged; a root replica is ankylosed to bone, onto which a restoration is placed. This will mean the implant restoration will function in a unique fashion under load. It is important to

S. Davies (✉)
Division of Dentistry, University of Manchester, Manchester, UK
e-mail: stephen.j.davies@manchester.ac.uk

P. Young
Oral Surgery, Northwich, Cheshire, UK
e-mail: peter.young@oralimplants.co.uk

A. Aminian
Private Practice, Wilmslow, UK
e-mail: Amin@clinic334.co.uk



C. Barclay (ed.), *Oral Implantology: Assessment to Maintenance*, BDJ Clinician's Guides, https://doi.org/10.1007/978-3-031-55241-0_8

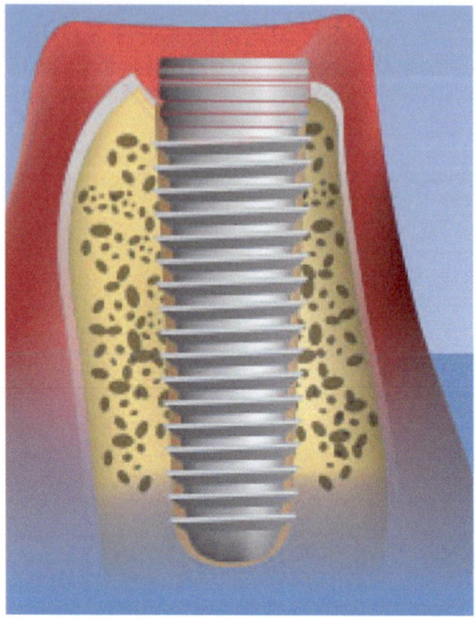

**Fig. 8.1** A dental implant anchored in bone

understand how the implant-supported restoration performs and where the biomechanics will differ from the performance of a tooth-supported restoration.

Regardless of analogue or digital approaches to care, a dental implant is simply a precisely engineered unit acting as a root replacement, with an absence of periodontal ligament and other features outlined in Fig. 8.1. A misunderstanding or a lack of appreciation of the the unique biomechanics of a dental implant may lead to a range of avoidable complications and ultimately restoration failure. Occlusal considerations are a fundamental component of this biomechanical performance.

Biomechanics has been defined as the structure, function and motion of the mechanical aspects of biological systems [3]. Understanding biomechanics is an important aspect of providing any dental restorations, where it is suggested that the biology "drives" the mechanics with a tooth-borne restoration. With an implant restoration, however, it is the mechanics that "drive", or promote, and maintain the biology.

Understanding the biomechanical performance of the implant-borne prosthesis plays an important role in the decision-making process when planning every aspect of the implant restoration (Table 8.1).

## 8.2 Understanding the Fundamentals of Implant Restoration Biomechanics

The connection of the prosthesis to the implant is reliant on engineering principles, with the aim of providing a compatible biomechanical unit with precise and intimal connections. Biomechanical principles also apply to the tooth-borne restoration (Fig. 8.2), where overloading of the restoration will result in one or any combination of complications, as the "biology drives the mechanics":

**Table 8.1** Factors to consider when planning an implant restoration

| Factors |
|---|
| Occlusal design (including guidance, management of patients with parafunction, occlusal surface area) |
| Restorative material |
| Stability/nature of opposing contacts |
| Implant restoration (fixed or removable) |
| Adjacent and opposing dentition stability (ranging from no mobility to fremitus, to mobile teeth) |
| Occlusal surface area of restoration |
| Screw vs. cement-retained fixed restorations |
| Abutment choice (angulation, material) |
| Angle correction |
| Cement choice for cement-retained restorations |
| Passivity of fit |
| Implications of cantilevered pontics |
| Implant connection design (internal vs. external connection), including platform switching |
| Implant dimensions (height and width) |
| Inter-occlusal distance |
| Loading protocols (immediate vs. delayed) |
| Splinted vs. un-splinted adjacent crowns |
| Axial vs non-axial loading |
| Conventional straight-line access vs. co-axial screw access designs |
| Cross-arch bracing |
| Implant-to-tooth connection with bridgework |
| Extent and status of denture-bearing area, for removable prostheses |

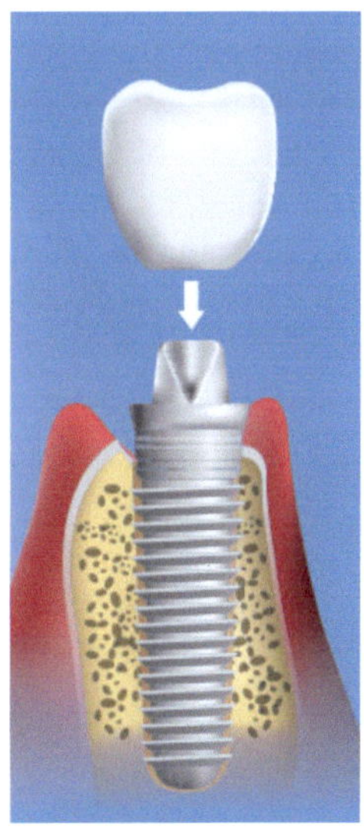

**Fig. 8.2** A crown on a dental implant abutment

- Fremitus/hypermobility
- Orthodontic movement
- Thickening of the periodontal ligament
- Tactile sensitivity

- Proprioception from periodontal ligament and pulp
- Pain

Biomechanics also plays a role in the occlusal performance of the implant-borne restoration, irrespective of whether fixed or removable, but with fundamental differences from the tooth-borne restoration:

- No tactile perception
- No periodontal ligament
- Stress concentration at crest of ridge (compared to periodontal ligament in a natural tooth)

These were clearly described by Kim et al. [4]. Kim goes on to explain that these factors risk the occlusal overloading of implant restorations, and this in turn may lead to early implant failure. To mitigate these effects, increased support areas, an appreciation of proper force direction and reduction of force magnification are required. Furthermore, one must appreciate the dynamic, changing nature of occlusion and the need to re-evaluate and adjust implant occlusion on a regular basis.

In appreciating the importance of the mechanical "driver" of the biomechanical performance of an implant restoration, risk of predictable failures, including screw loosening, screw fracture, loss of integration, porcelain/material fracture, cement failure, can be reduced.

Attempts have been made to replicate the stress distribution properties of the periodontal ligament with dental implants incorporating movable components [5], but these have largely proven to be unsuccessful [6] (Fig. 8.3)

The aim of this chapter is to focus on the occlusal management of implant restoration and, for the sake of simplicity, will focus on fixed restoration. An understanding of occlusion in implant dentistry is relevant to the general dental practitioner, as they may be exposed to implant restorations either directly or indirectly:

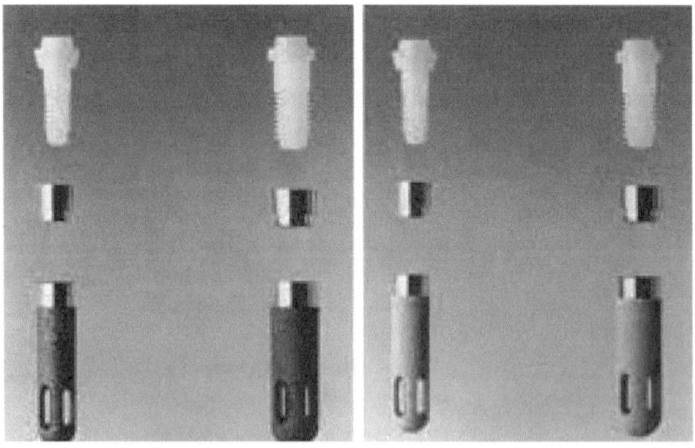

**Fig. 8.3** IMZ implant with intra-mobile element to simulate a periodontal ligament

- The clinician may incorporate implant dentistry (surgical +/− restorative aspects) into their working practice, as implants become an increasingly popular choice for patients considering replacement of missing/failing teeth.
- The clinician may not be interested in providing any aspect of implant care, but may be carrying out restoration of the opposing dentition to a pre-existing implant prosthesis. It is equally important to appreciate the biomechanical performance of the opposing units as a functioning pair.
- The clinician may be seeing the patient for the first time, presenting with complications due to occlusal issues (e.g., restoration de-bond, screw loosening, screw fracture, amongst others). The diagnosis and management may be carried out by the attending clinician, without the patient having the inconvenience or costs incurred with a referral. The immediate management of any complication is often critical, and re-cementing a restoration with definitive cements, or re-tightening a screw without following correct protocols may lead to potentially catastrophic consequences for the restoration. (Fig. 8.4).
- The clinician may be carrying out long-term care of the patient who has undergone implant treatment, where their dentition is likely to undergo changes (including wear, tooth migration), resulting in occlusal changes, which will have an impact on the biomechanical performance of the implant restoration over time.

This latter point is particularly important for all restorative clinicians, whether they plan to restore implants or not. Often Implant treatment is provided in a mouth that has experienced restorative challenges, failure and/or disease. The mouth and

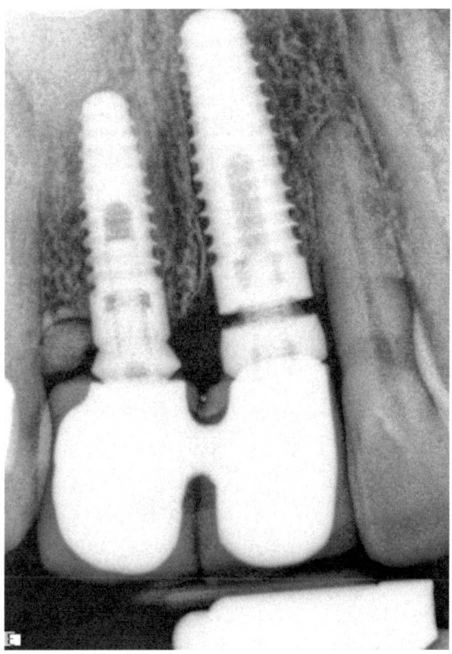

**Fig. 8.4** The patient was attended by an inexperienced dentist for re-cementation of the de-bonded implant crown. There is now excess cement in the peri-implant tissues, incomplete seating of the crowns and undiagnosed screw loosening on left implant. As expected, significant adjustment had to be made by the dentist upon checking the occlusion due to excessively high position of the restoration

dentition will change over time, leading to a different environment from the one planned for at the time of restoration delivery. These changes may involve not only teeth adjacent to and opposing the implant restoration, but also changes in the dentition distant to the implant restoration; all of these changes might impact the biomechanical loading of the implant. This will be discussed in further detail later in this chapter.

A theoretical "ideal" starting point for an implant restoration is for it to be placed in a well-maintained, healthy, stable and comfortable mouth with the appropriate number and position of implant(s) for the planned restoration(s), restored using the correct protocols, with stable adjacent and opposing units. The responsibility then falls on the patient and clinicians carrying out the long-term care to maintain, preserve and protect this "ideal' from the time of delivery throughout the long-term lifespan of the restoration. We intentionally use the term "clinicians", as the responsibility for the long-term care and monitoring of the implant-restored dentition is likely to fall on several clinicians over the lifetime of the patient, not forgetting the importance of the patient's role in maintaining day-to-day health.

## 8.3 Occlusal Management of the Implant Patient

We will proceed with discussing the occlusal management of the implant patient in three distinct phases of care:

1. Planning stage
2. Treatment stage, leading to restoration delivery
3. Short- and long-term management after restoration delivery

### 8.3.1 Planning Stage

Missing teeth, as a consequence of hypodontia, can be replaced with implant restorations, often as part of a multi-disciplinary approach. More commonly, implant treatment is used to replace teeth that are due to be extracted, or are missing as a consequence of disease, failure (mechanical/structural) or trauma (occlusal or impact). The reasons for the failure of an implant restoration may fall into categories similar to those of tooth-borne restorations, and identifying the risk factors is an important aspect of the diagnostic stage of care. The occlusal factors that contributed to the failure of the original teeth/restorations may also cause the failure of implant restorations, with the obvious exceptions of dental caries and resorption.

Removing, or at least controlling, the risk factors will have a significant impact on success. The risk of an implant restoration failing as a result of excessive/uncontrolled contacts with its counterpart can be termed as occlusal risk and is one of the parameters to be assessed at the outset.

Assessment should examine and record the number (quantitative) and degree/position/stability (qualitative aspects) of occlusal contacts, before commencement of treatment:

- Tooth contacts in static occlusion
- Posterior support
- Number of occluding units
- Stability of anterior and posterior contacts
- Locked occlusion (i.e a lack of Freedom in Centric Occlusion, in both anterior and posterior segments)
- Dynamic occlusion (or articulation) and guidance/nature of guidance in protrusion and lateral excursive movements
- Presence or absence of working and non-working side interferences and their impact on implant restoration.
- Status of teeth/restorations providing guiding contacts (heavily restored, root-treated +/− posts)
- Features of any form of tooth surface loss, particularly parafunction
- Fremitus/hypermobility

The occlusal assessment should not only include the above features at the time of presentation, but also plan for how they are expected to evolve from the pre-treatment phase, during treatment and into the post-treatment phase. As an example, removal of failed/failing teeth that are planned for implant replacement may create a change in guidance after their extraction. The tooth/teeth now providing the guidance may have a compromised structure (root-treated either with or without post support, large direct restoration without cuspal coverage) and may be at increased risk of failing during treatment, or in the early and unexpected phase after treatment. This is considered poor planning.

Figure 8.5 shows the dental panoramic tomogram/orthopantomograph (DPT/OPG) of a patient looking for treatment options for the missing teeth in the

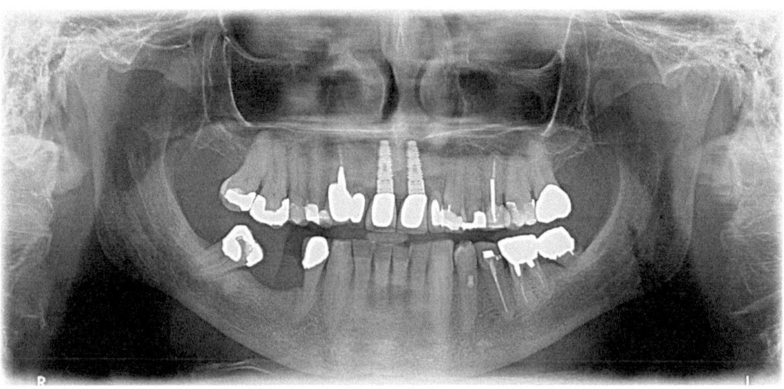

**Fig. 8.5** Patient looking for treatment options for the missing teeth in the lower-right quadrant

lower-right quadrant. He had been provided with a post-retained bridge, placed on the maxillary right canine 20+ years ago. Assessment confirmed occlusal protection of the bridge was provided by the working side interference from the lower right molar, i.e., only light contacts in centric/inter-cuspal position were noted on the canine, with no contacts on excursive movements. Any treatment of the molar (from provision of direct or indirect restoration, or extraction) is likely to alter its occlusal scheme with the consequence of removing protection of the canine abutment, leading to a likely catastrophic failure of the bridge. The planning process meant the patient was made aware that complex treatment would be needed at some point in the future, either for provision of a full-coverage crown for the heavily restored lower molar (to copy the excursive guidance) or implant replacement of the canine bridge. In the meantime, continued protection from the lower molar would have to be monitored and maintained. The discussions at the planning stage did not, therefore, solely focus on the missing units and their replacement options.

### 8.3.2 Treatment Stage

Occlusal control during treatment is necessary to ensure that any stability identified at the planning stage is maintained. It is also during this phase that occlusal stability may be introduced in anticipation of the planned restorations, including space creation for the final restoration. Figure 8.6 show porcelain fracture experienced on the implant crown because of a change in the occlusion, resulting in an overload of the material. The placement of direct composite on the palatal aspect of the natural canine teeth imparted steeper canine guidance, leading to a larger restorative space for the replacement restorations, allowing for aesthetics to be restored.

It is also during this stage that any lack of inter-occlusal space identified at the planning stage can be addressed. This may be with orthodontic intrusion (Fig. 8.7) or restorative techniques. The use of direct composite restorations in the management of tooth surface loss can also be directed towards space creation. This may be as simple as providing a composite canine riser to increase the inter-occlusal space

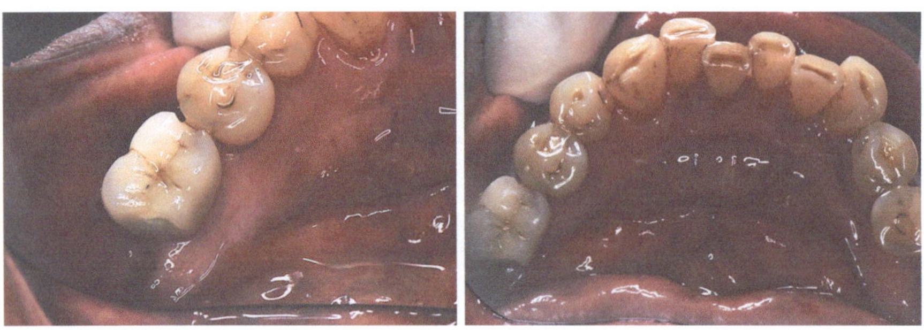

**Fig. 8.6** Ceramic fracture on implant crown. Note wear on natural teeth and minor crowding. Both changes, over the course of years, are likely to have resulted in an unplanned change in occlusal loading of the implant crown, leading to ceramic fracture complication

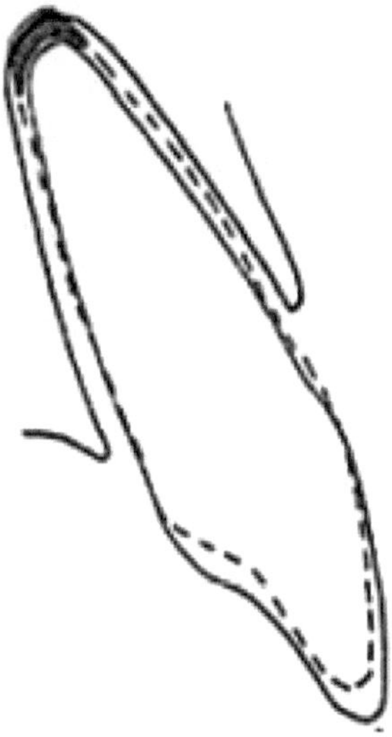

**Fig. 8.7** Orthodontic intrusion

on dynamic excursions (Fig. 8.8) or may necessitate a more comprehensive full-mouth approach.

Figure 8.9 demonstrates the case series of a 65-year-old patient looking for replacement of missing teeth to improve function. The patient opted for treatment of only the upper left side, but insufficient space for restoration indicated the placement of composite resin build-ups for a conservative approach to increase the occlusal vertical dimension (OVD). Building up the worn upper arch only would mean there would still not be sufficient space for the implant restorations. Direct composite resin was therefore placed on the palatal aspect of the maxillary anteriors and facial/incisal aspect of the mandibular anteriors, to create the required space. This is shown in Fig. 8.10.

#### 8.3.2.1 Restoration Design and Fit

The single-unit restoration or short-span bridgework can be used to discuss the basic requirements when designing and delivering an implant borne restoration. The biomechanical performance of the restoration will change depending on the extent of the restoration and also the nature of the opposing arch, be it a completely removable denture, a fully dentate and stable arch or a fixed full-arch implant reconstruction. The latter, in particular, creates its own dynamic that has to be considered when two opposing implant restorations are provided.

For the sake of simplicity, we will consider the provision a single tooth implant restoration against an opposing arch that is intact, stable, and healthy with no teeth showing any significant mobility. The implant restoration should have the following prescription provided for the laboratory technician, or incorporated into the design should a digital process be implemented:

- Flat occlusal platform (i.e., no exaggerated occlusal anatomy)

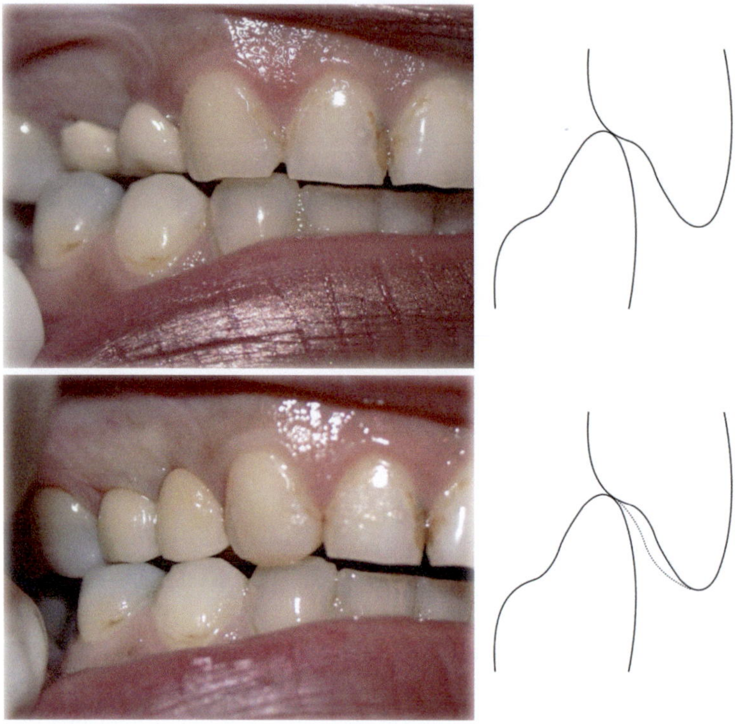

**Fig. 8.8** Composite canine riser to increase palatal ramp and create greater inter-occlusal space on dynamic movements

- Broad contact area
- Shallow guidance angle
- No sole contribution to working or non-working side interferences
- Ideally avoiding being the sole guidance surface in any part of excursive movements
- Narrow occlusal platform

On fitting the restoration, whether cement or screw-retained, the occlusal features prescribed are checked on the model before transferring to the mouth. A quantitative assessment of the occlusal contacts can be carried out with thin coloured articulating paper. This is carried out before and after restoration fit to confirm no changes have been introduced. A qualitative look at the contact on the implant restoration can then be carried out using a shimstock foil. The shipstock foil shuld now be trapped between all the contacting natural teeth. This is due to the compression of the periodontium that can occur in natural teeth; no such movement is possible in the implant supported restoration. It should be possible to remove the foil, with slight resistance created by the contacting units. The exercise is repeated with the patient being asked to close firmly. The movement of all the contacting natural teeth

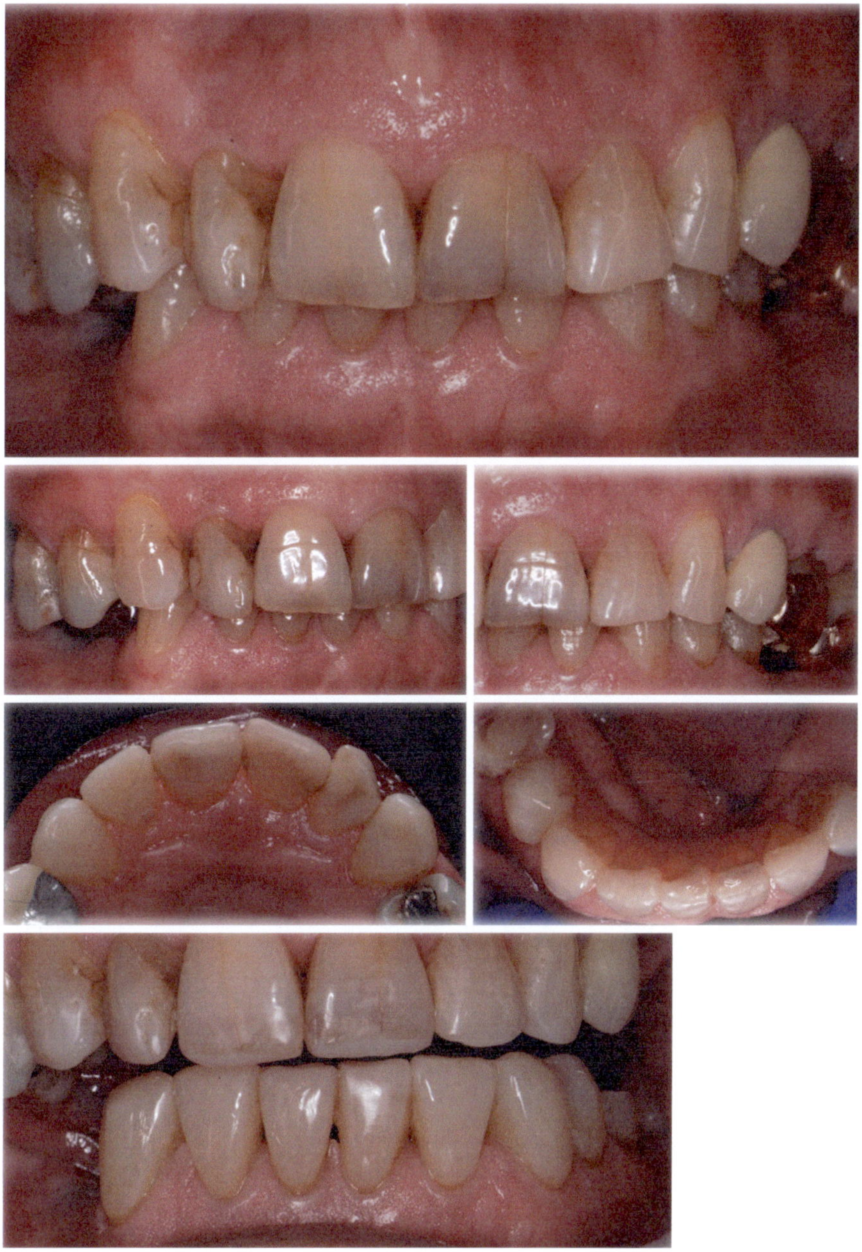

**Fig. 8.9** Demonstrates the case series of a 65-year-old patient looking for replacement of missing teeth to improve function

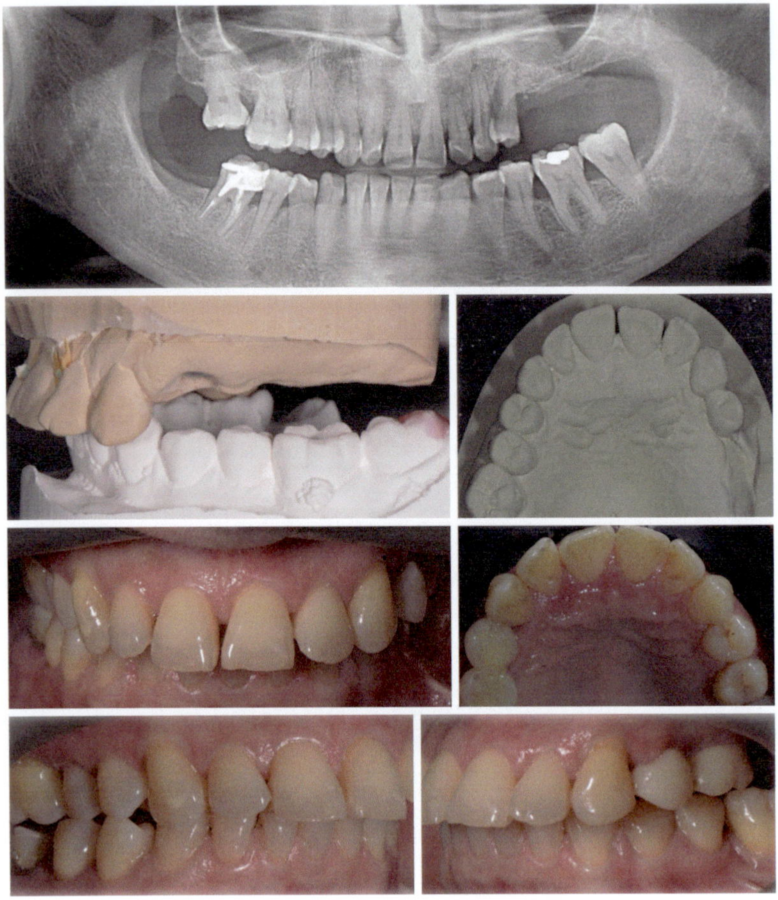

**Fig. 8.10** Cases series photographs of full-mouth approach to increase OVD and create inter-occlusal space for restorations in the upper-left quadrant

in the periodontium, with no movement in the implant restoration, should lead to trapping of the foil (Fig. 8.11).

A clinician may have no experience or interest in providing implant treatment but may be restoring a tooth that opposes a fixed implant crown or bridge. The same considerations need to be taken into account when fitting this restoration.

### 8.3.3 Occlusal Management Post-Treatment

The endpoint of the restorative phase should aim for a completed implant restoration with optimal fit in a stable, healthy mouth with a protected occlusal scheme. The aim of the post-restorative phase is to monitor, protect and maintain this environment, accepting that changes are inevitable.

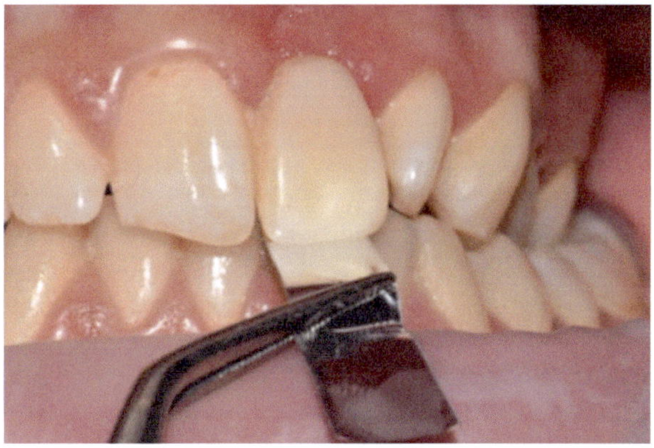

**Fig. 8.11** Use of shimstock when checking occlusal contacts (this image needs replacing)

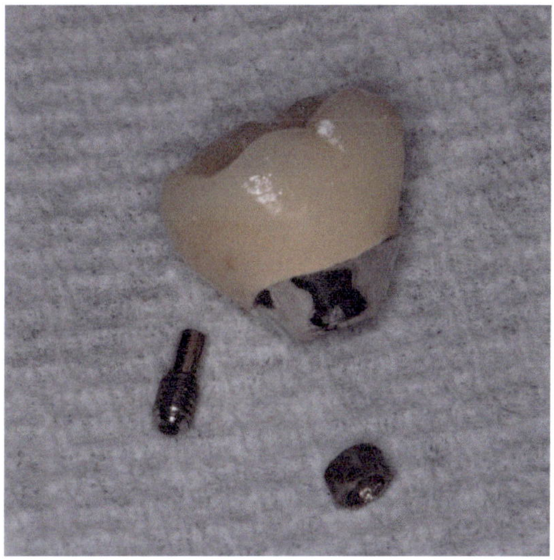

**Fig. 8.12** Abutment and screw fracture because of possible occlusal overload

There may be several reasons leading to occlusal changes, which create altered loading of the fixed implant restoration:

- Tooth wear of the natural teeth, albeit these will be very gradual changes. Tooth surface loss induced changes in the occlusion may also occur relatively soon after restoration delivery, leading to failure (Fig. 8.12).
- Wear of restorative materials over time. This will be expected in cases of tooth-surface loss that are restored with direct composite. The build-ups would be expected to chip or wear (cohesive failure) over time. They may also de-bond (adhesive failure), although this risk should be minimised with good bonding protocol and where there is sufficient available enamel for a bonding interface. This risk can be minimised with splint wear and regular monitoring.

- Restoration of teeth with direct and indirect procedures leading to changes in the occlusion.
- Migration of the natural teeth, either through compensatory movements or elective orthodontics. Open contact areas which develop between implant restorations and adjacent teeth, over the course of years, confirm migration of the natural dentition.
- Loss and non-replacement of teeth or failed restorations, leading to an increased load on the remaining teeth and restorations.
- Loss of teeth or failed restorations and replacement with mucosal-supported removable prostheses, leading to an increased load on the remaining teeth and restorations.
- The number of teeth may remain unchanged, but changes in occlusal loading over time may lead to fremitus, presenting as slight mobility of certain teeth. This is likely to lead to changes in the type and magnitude of occlusal forces on the remaining teeth and, in particular, rigid implant restorations.
- The number of teeth may remain unchanged, but changes in bone support over time may lead to increased mobility. Again, this is likely to lead to changes in the type and magnitude of the occlusal forces on the remaining teeth and restorations.

Any unexpected change in the loading is likely to be, by definition, unintended, unpredictable and probably detrimental to the implant restoration. Most changes are likely to be gradual, leading to progressive altered and/or over-loading of the implant restoration, with presentation of complications over the course of years. Other changes may be more sudden, such as loss of teeth.

The long-term monitoring of occlusal loading of the fixed-implant restoration is an important aspect of maintenance. All patients who have undergone implant treatment, by virtue of having this treatment, are considered as at-risk of periodontitis/peri-implant tissue disease. This risk is exaggerated should they have experienced any form of severe periodontal disease. This risk is identified at the outset, with the patient being informed. The risk is minimised with a regular hygiene and maintenance programme implemented before treatment, and continued throughout and after treatment. Similarly, patients considering implant treatment may have signs of tooth-surface loss at the planning stage and can be considered as being in the "occlusal risk" category (Fig. 8.13). A regime of close monitoring and prevention (probable splint wear) should be highlighted at the outset. It is suggested that as part of the consent process, that the need to follow the failure preventative protocols, which may include splint wearing, are explicit; then any unexpected failures due to patient's deviation from their preventative protocol is their cost.

In summary, the placement of an implant restoration increases the occlusal risk status of that patient's dentition, meaning there is an increased emphasis on careful case selection, planning and execution of treatment. The process will allow for the risk factors for failure to be identified and ideally removed. In most cases, however, the risk can only be reduced or controlled through long-term maintenance and monitoring, making these aspects fundamental to a predictable outcome. The

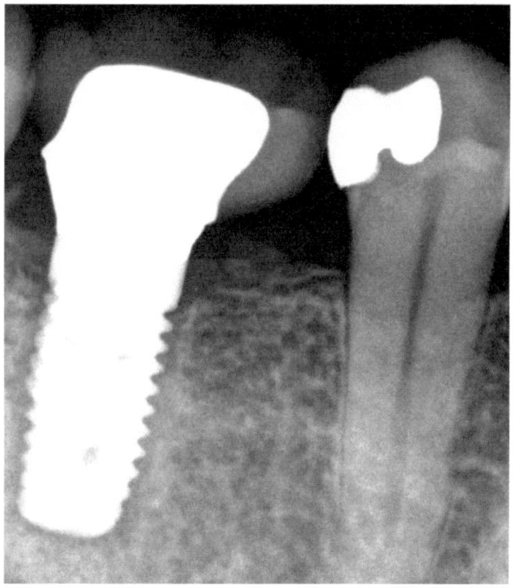

**Fig. 8.13** The loss of implant/bone contact and therefore implant failure

importance of identifying, removing, controlling/minimising and monitoring the occlusal risks should not be underestimated, and this responsibility may fall on a clinician who is not involved in the initial phase of treatment. Any occlusal stability that is achieved at the time of restoration delivery is likely to be challenged with changes in the patient's natural dentition (wear, extractions, mobility, migration) and provision of restorations. It is for this reason that the authors believe all dental practitioners should have a good understanding of the role of biomechanics and occlusion in the success of implant treatment.

## References


1. Adell R, Lekholm U, Rockler B, Brånemark PI. A 15-year study of osseointegrated implants in the treatment of the edentulous jaw. Int J Oral Surg. 1981;10(6):387–416. https://doi.org/10.1016/s0300-9785(81)80077-4. PubMed PMID: 6809663.
2. Brånemark PI, Adell R, Breine U, Hansson BO, Lindström J, Ohlsson A. Intra-osseous anchorage of dental prostheses. I. Experimental studies. Scand J Plast Reconstr Surg. 1969;3(2):81–100. https://doi.org/10.3109/02844316909036699. PubMed PMID: 4924041.
3. Oxford English Dictionary. Oxford University Press. biomechanics, n.
4. Kim Y, Oh TJ, Misch CE, Wang HL. Occlusal considerations in implant therapy: clinical guidelines with biomechanical rationale. Clin Oral Implants Res. 2005;16(1):26–35. https://doi.org/10.1111/j.1600-0501.2004.01067.x. PubMed PMID: 15642028.
5. Babbush CA, Kirsch A, Mentag PJ, Hill B. Intramobile cylinder (IMZ) two-stage osteointegrated implant system with the intramobile element (IME): part I. Its ratinale and procedure for use. Int J Oral Maxillofac Implants. 1987;2(4):203–16. PubMed PMID: 3333644.
6. Kirsch A, Ackermann KL. The IMZ osteointegrated implant system. Dent Clin N Am. 1989;33(4):733–91.

# Implant Maintenance and Aftercare

# 9

Craig Barclay

As increasing number of dental implants are being placed in the general population, the need to develop a maintenance protocol that caters to the needs of the patients has become essential. Historically, dental implants were predominantly placed in the early edentulous population; however, the shift of placements to the wider population means that a patient-focused approach to peri-implant maintenance therapy (PIMT) and the effect this has on biological complications and implant survival need to be considered. This has been considered in the new periodontal classification (2017), which includes peri-implant diseases and conditions for the first time. Lang et al. [1] discussed Cumulative Interceptive Therapy (CIST), which suggested that the prevention of implant disease was better than the management of the disease itself. However, it is crucial to acknowledge that implant disease does not arise purely from microbes and the body's inflammatory response to them. As stated by Albrektsson and his colleagues, there are numerous additional factors that contribute to implant failure and disease, encompassing various clinical and patient-related factors. Clearly, it is imperative that we educate our implant patients on how to clean their implant superstructures and abutments; however, as clinicians, we need to be cognizant of the fact that the pellicle that develops on titanium, either the implant surface itself or the implant abutment, differs from that which develops on enamel and cementum. In 1996, Edgerton demonstrated that a high molecular weight proline rich glycoprotein pellicle forms on the dental implants, and this may contribute to the difference in the adhesion rates of the pellicles and also the type of specific bacteria found in implant crevices and surfaces.

Some authors differentiate between primary peri-implantitis, where the sole cause of bone loss is the bacterial infection itself, and secondary peri-implantitis, where the bacterial infection is secondary to another underlying issue that is causing bone loss. (Table 9.1).

C. Barclay (✉)
Restorative Dentistry/Oral Rehabilitation, Manchester Foundation Trust, Manchester, UK
e-mail: craig.barclay@mft.nhs.uk



C. Barclay (ed.), *Oral Implantology: Assessment to Maintenance*, BDJ Clinician's Guides, https://doi.org/10.1007/978-3-031-55241-0_9

**Table 9.1** Suggested causes of variation in bone loss around implants

| |
|---|
| Bacterial infection caused by excess plaque build-up. |
| The effects of smoking |
| The microgap |
| The biological width concept |
| Clinical plaque formation in relation to surface roughness |
| The hypothesis of reduced peri-implant bone loss for platform-switched implants |
| Occlusal overloading being an important cause for marginal bone resorption |
| The observation of marginal bone loss being influenced by certain implant designs |
| The observation of a coupling between clinical handling and bone resorption |
| Patient related factors contributing to marginal bone loss |
| Excess cement and risks for marginal bone loss |

Implant health would be considered as being the absence of clinical signs of inflammation, the absence of bleeding and/or suppuration, no increase in probing depths and the absence of bone loss at the crestal level from a baseline radiograph.

From a diagnostic standpoint, clinical challenges may arise when probing around implants due to inherent inaccuracies. This can be due to the probing pressure used to assess pocket depths being reduced in comparison to that used to probe around natural teeth. This can be as a result of the gingival attachment mechanisms around dental implants. Other issues include difficulties with probe adaptation around a dental implant, particularly in platform-switched dental implant connections and, finally, depending on the degree of inflammation, penetration of the probe may vary.

Similarly, when it comes to radiographic diagnosis, this can also prove challenging. This may be due to the time intervals between radiographs, the angulation of the 2D film, potential lack of baseline comparison, and finally, if 3D imaging is used, the scatter/beam hardening.

## 9.1 What Should We Advise in Terms of Patient Hygiene Measures Around Their Dental Implants?

It is imperative that we educate our patients that maintaining dental implants is as important as looking after natural teeth. Although, clearly, dental implants cannot suffer from caries, the understanding of the detrimental effects of plaque around a dental implant is crucial. In 1986, Quirynen discussed the anatomical and inflammatory factors that influence bacterial growth and retention in humans, demonstrating that plaque grows faster on a titanium surface compared to enamel. Therefore, it is essential to stress the importance of effective plaque removal around dental implants and their superstructure [2]. The potential consequences can be seen in Figs. 9.1 and 9.2.

Scientific literature has investigated whether using an electric toothbrush is more effective compared to a manual toothbrush, and the findings suggest that an electric toothbrush tends to be more effective.

A Cochrane review suggested a 21% reduction in plaque with powered toothbrushes compared to manual toothbrushes. Ensuring that a correct and consistent

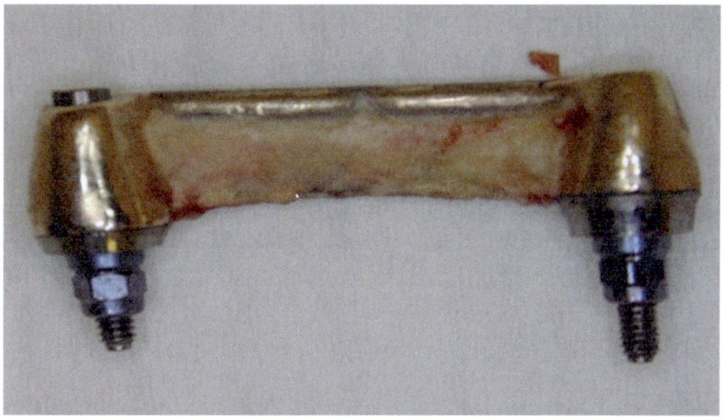

**Fig. 9.1** Plaque and calculus adherant to a dental implant bar

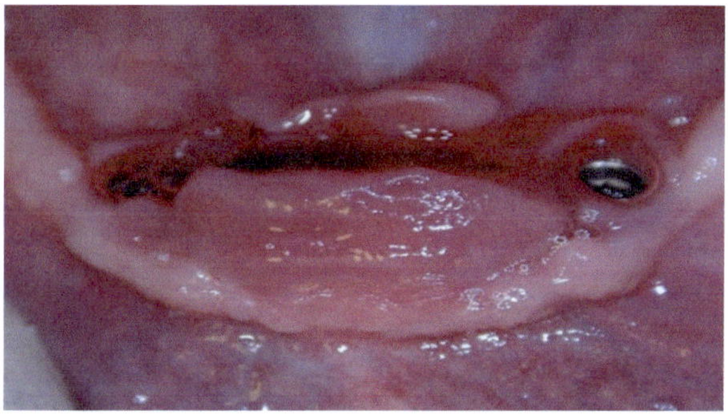

**Fig. 9.2** The corresponding soft tissue inflammation as a result of the palque and calculus

approach to plaque removal is likely as important as the choice of tool used for plaque removal.

Whether the surface roughness of the implant itself or the collar affects plaque adherence has been investigated by Quirynen and colleagues [3]. Their research exchanged the abutments on clinically osseo-integrated implants with a rougher type, and reported that only minor differences in the macroscopical plaque were noticed, quantitatively and qualitatively. Wennerberg et al. performed a similar study, in which they found no correlation between plaque formation and the roughness of abutments [4]; however, they did note that there was a clear individual patient pattern in the amount of plaque formed on the implant abutment. Finally, Baldi et al. reported greater plaque accumulation on dual-acid-etched surfaces compared with machined surfaces. However, they also noted that these dual-acid-etched surfaces displayed significantly less marginal bone loss than the machined ones.

It is, therefore, accepted that surface chemistry and the design features of an implant abutment or collar play a significant role in biofilm formation due to surface-free energy. Edgerton et al. [5] found that the pellicle present on the titanium surface consisted of cystatins and low-molecular-weight mucin, as compared to a high-molecular-weight proline-rich glycoprotein found on enamel surfaces Fig. 9.3 and 9.4.

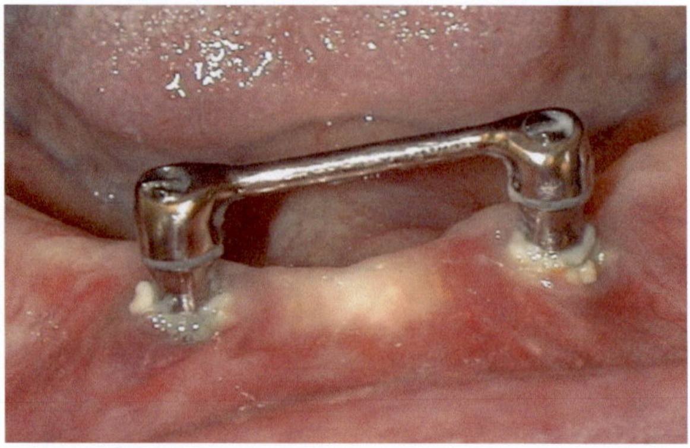

**Fig. 9.3** Plaque and calculus adherence to an old IMZ implant surface, resulting in its exfoliation

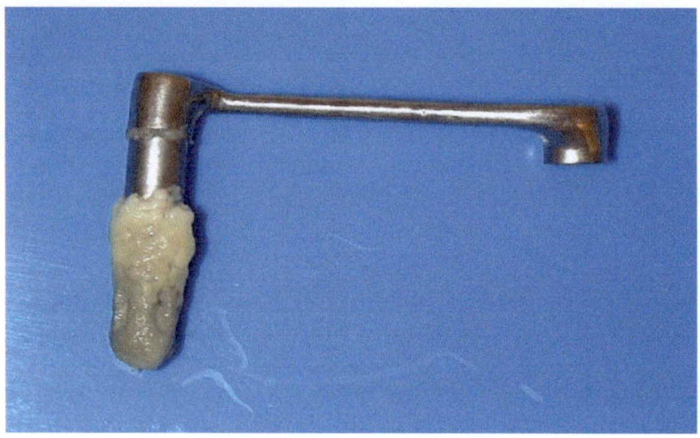

**Fig. 9.4** Plaque and calculus adherence to an old IMZ implant surface, resulting in its exfoliation

## 9.2 Should Patients Be Advised to Floss Around Their Dental Implants?

There are several hypothetical concerns raised regarding flossing around dental implants:

- The soft tissue around a dental implant is less well-innervated than that around a tooth; therefore, the sensation of pain due to incorrect flossing may not deter a patient in the same way as it may around a natural tooth.
- The issue of platform-switching and the emergence profile of the implant superstructure may make flossing problematic and may lead to floss threading and remnants of floss remaining in the soft tissues around a dental implant. Considering this, flossing around dental implants should be done with extreme caution, and patients should be instructed to never push the floss down into the gingival pocket. If they are unable to floss around the restoration without disturbing the peri-implant seal, it is best to simply not floss around the implant at all.

Hence, although lacking robust scientific evidence, Lang [6] and other researchers have suggested the potential harm of flossing around dental implants.

Use of interdental brushes was investigated as early as 1976 [7], when it was found that they were effective in removing plaque as far as 2–2.5 mm below the gingival margin. Subsequently, the European Federation of Periodontology, in 2015, demonstrated that "cleaning with interdental brushes is the most effective method for interproximal plaque removal, consistently associated with more plaque removal than flossing or woodsticks". Finally, Chongcharoen showed the effectiveness of different interdental brushes in cleaning the interproximal surfaces of teeth and implants in a randomized, controlled, double-blind cross-over study [8]. It is, therefore, important that an interdental brush with the correct size and shape is demonstrated to the patient for use around dental implants [9, 10].

## 9.3 What Should We Advise Regarding the Use of Irrigation Devices Around Dental Implants?

The use of oral irrigators for implant maintenance was shown by Magnuson et al., who observed that the water flosser group had significantly greater bleeding reduction than the group that carried out floss cleaning around implants. A randomized controlled study by Bunk [11] showed that within the limits of the study, adjuvant use of an oral irrigator with 0.06% Chlorhexidine (CHX) in addition to mechanical biofilm removal and oral hygiene instruction can reduce the presence and severity of peri-implant mucositis after 12 weeks of use. Other studies have shown that the use of oral irrigators can significantly improve biofilm removal.

It is, therefore, suggested that the adjunctive use of an oral irrigator with either chlorhexidine or Listerine aids the removal of biofilm and plaque interproximally around dental implants.

## 9.4 The Importance of Attached/Keratinized Mucosa Around the Implant Collar

Many studies have shown that the amount of soft-tissue recession was significantly increased at implant sites with narrow keratinized mucosa, but the amount of keratinized mucosa had little effect on deepening of the peri-implant pockets. The evidence related to the effect of keratinized mucosa on the changes of attachment or bone levels is limited, and conclusions could not be drawn at present. In addition, Ravida found that a band of keratinized mucosa [12] was not absolutely necessary for the maintenance of peri-implant tissue, whereas lack of adequate keratinized mucosa around the implant might impede proper oral hygiene performance and compromise the aesthetic results.

A systematic review by Ravida included nine studies investigating the effect of the presence or absence of sufficient amount of keratinized tissue around dental implants on peri-implant tissue health [13]. The results of the meta-analysis concluded that the presence of sufficient amount of keratinized tissue is associated with less plaque accumulation, gingival inflammation, recession and less bone loss. However, no significant difference was found regarding bleeding on probing (BOP), plaque index (PI), and probing depth (PD). Further, future standardized studies are needed to determine the clinical significance of keratinized tissue around dental implants, as there are still many disagreements in the literature; however, it is generally accepted that for a patient to be able to clean effectively around a dental implant a collar of keratinized mucosa is preferable.

## 9.5 The Importance of Probing Around Implants to Assess Dental Implant Health

Recording pocket depths around dental implants cannot be performed in the same way as recording pocket depths around natural teeth. Dental implants do not have a cementum layer covering their surface, and thus a soft-tissue attachment similar to a tooth does not exist. Although collagen fibre bundles are present in the implant soft tissue, they originate from the bone surface and run vertically and parallel to the implant surface itself. Also, if a platform switch has occurred, the shape of this junction between a dental implant and the abutment/crown may not lend itself to conventional dental probing.

Coli et al. suggested guarded processing of bleeding on probing data around dental implants [14], as this may be due to disruption of the fragile soft-tissue architecture around the implant collar, as opposed to marginal bone loss and inflammation. The question of whether to probe around a dental implant is a difficult one, but clearly observation of the tissue to see if the peri-implant mucosa is inflamed or indeed if there is any exudate from the soft tissues is essential to monitor gingival health (Fig. 9.5).

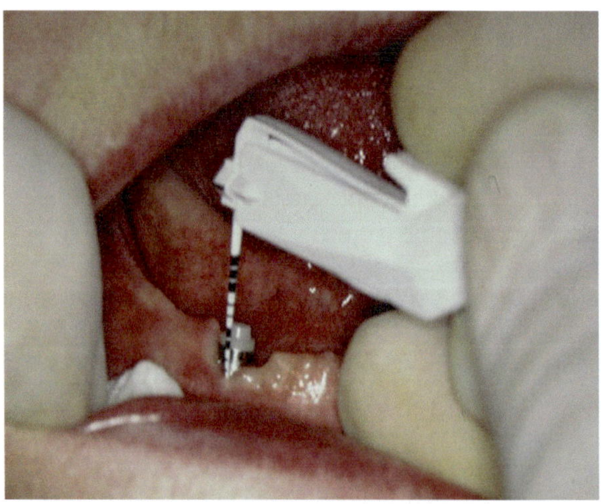

**Fig. 9.5** Probing around a dental implant

## 9.6 The Importance of Albrektsson Bone Loss Criteria in Implant Maintenance

Albrektsson et al. claimed that the bone loss was <0.2 mm annually after the 1 year of prosthetic loading in successful cases [15]. He also showed that, for newer implant surfaces, you should expect no more than 1 mm of coronal bone loss within the first year; this suggests that physiological bone loss around an implant over time is acceptable as long as it is within the permissible limits. Clearly, a dental implant would be considered to be failing if it shows a peri-implant bone loss of greater than 1.0 mm in the first year and greater than 0.2 mm per year thereafter. It is important to appreciate the difference between physiological bone loss around a dental implant and pathological bone loss. It is also important to determine whether the pathological bone loss is an acute or chronic a condition, as this will affect how you would consider maintaining the dental implant and managing the disease process.

## References


1. Lang NP, Wilson TG, Corbett. Biological complications with dental implants: their prevention, diagnosis and treatment. EF Clin Oral Impl Res. 2000;11:146–55.
2. Chapple IL, Van der Weijden F, Doerfer C, Herrera D, Shapira L, Polak D, Madianos P, Louropoulou A, Machtei E, Donos N, et al. Primary prevention of periodontitis: managing gingivitis. J Clin Periodontol. 2015;42(Suppl. 16):S71–6.
3. Quirynen M, De Soete M, van Steenberghe D. Infectious risks for oral implants: a review of the literature. Clin Oral Implants Res. 2002;13(1):1–19. https://doi.org/10.1034/j.16000501.2002.130101.x.
4. Wennerberg A, Albrektsson T, Andersson B. Design and surface characteristics of 13 commercially available oral implant systems. Int J Oral Maxillofac Implants. 1993;8:622–33.
5. Edgerton M, Lo SE, Scannapieco FA. Experimental salivary pellicles formed on titanium surfaces mediate adhesion of streptococci. Int J Oral Maxillofac Implants. 1996;11(4):443–9.
6. Lang NP, Schulten EAJM, Christiaan M. Dental floss as a possible risk for the development of peri-implant disease: an observational study of 10 cases. Clin Oral Implants Res. 2015;27:618–21.
7. Waerhaug J. The interdental brush and its place in operative and crown and bridge dentistry. J Oral Rehabil. 1976;3:107–13. https://doi.org/10.1111/j.1365-2842.
8. Chongcharoen N, Lulic M, Lang NP. Effectiveness of different interdental brushes on cleaning the interproximal surfaces of teeth and implants: a randomized controlled, double-blind cross-over study. Clin Oral Implants Res. 2012;23(5):635–40.
9. Magnuson B, Harsono M, Stark PC, Lyle D, Kugel G, Perry R. Comparison of the effect of two interdental cleaning devices around implants on the reduction of bleeding: a 30-day randomized clinical trial. Compend Contin Educ Dent. 2013;34:2–7.
10. Ng E, Lim LP. An overview of different interdental cleaning aids and their effectiveness. Dent J (Basel). 2019;7(2):56. https://doi.org/10.3390/dj7020056.
11. Bunk D, Eisenburger M, Häckl S, Eberhard J, Stiesch M, Grischke J. The effect of adjuvant oral irrigation on self-administered oral care in the management of peri-implant mucositis: a randomized controlled clinical trial. Clin Oral Impl Res. 2020;31:946–58.

12. Ravidà A, et al. The role of keratinized mucosa width as a risk factor for peri-implant disease: a systematic review, meta-analysis, and trial sequential analysis. Clin Implant Dent Relat Res. 2022;24(3):287–300.
13. Kamal RK. Necessity of keratinized tissue around dental implants to maintain peri-implant tissue health: a systematic review. Dental Theses. 2018, p. 33.
14. Coli P, Jemt T. Are marginal bone level changes around dental implants due to infection? Clin Implant Dent Relat Res. 2021;23:170–7.
15. Albrektsson T, Zarb G, Worthington P, Eriksson AR. The long-term efficacy of currently used dental implants: a review and proposed criteria of success. Int J Oral Maxillofac Implants. 1986;1:11–25.

# Managing Implant Repair, Problems and Failure

# 10

Nigel Saynor

## 10.1 Introduction

The survival of a dental implant relies on successful osseointegration following placement. The biological healing process may be adversely affected by excessive surgical trauma, infection and systemic disorders, thereby negatively affecting the outcome. When the implant is restored and placed into function, the bone remodelling process becomes a major factor and is critical to the survival of the implant.

One of the key issues faced by all implantologists today are the complications and failures occurring with the provision of dental implant treatment. To further optimise and improve new treatment outcomes, aetiologies and factors associated with dental implant failures and complications should be recognised. Conceivably, such knowledge is required for developing adequate treatment and prevention strategies.

Dental implants play a vital role in the rehabilitation of our patients with a variety of treatment modalities. Although the success rates are significantly high, failures do occur for a wide variety of reasons and can have devastating consequences.

Implant failure is the first instance at which the performance of the implant, measured in a quantitative way, falls below a specified and acceptable level.

Implant failure is defined as the total failure of the implant to fulfil its purpose (functional, aesthetic and phonetic) as a result of mechanical or biological reasons as well as an inadequacy of the host tissue to establish or maintain osseointegration.

N. Saynor (✉)
Bramcote Dental Practice, Bramhall, Stockport, UK



C. Barclay (ed.), *Oral Implantology: Assessment to Maintenance*, BDJ Clinician's Guides, https://doi.org/10.1007/978-3-031-55241-0_10

## 10.2 Defining Ailing, Failing, Failed and Surviving Implants

*Ailing Implants* is a term that was introduced to describe implants that are clinically affected by bone loss with pocketing but are stable. Their management can be seen in elsewhere in this text— in the section titled "Complication/Failure Management".

*Failing Implants* display features similar to those of ailing implants but are resistant to treatment and continue to deteriorate

*Failed Implant* is one that is clinically mobile, radiographically shows a generalised circumferential radiolucency or, has totally fractured. These implants require immediate removal to prevent further loss of osseous tissue.

*Surviving Implants*, a term described by Albrektsson, applies to implants that are functional, but not tested against success criteria.

## 10.3 Success and Failure Studies

Longitudinal studies have demonstrated that the success rates for maxillary implants range between 80% and 85% at the 10-year mark, whilst success rates for implants in the anterior mandible can be as high as 98%.

Despite the significant success rates, failures sadly do occur and can be devastating for patients; therefore, it is important to examine the failure rates within the literature. Esposito et al. reported a failure rate of 7.7% in a sample of 3000 dental implants at 5 years. Bain and May reported a 6% failure rate over a 6-year period in 540 patients with 2000 implants. Whilst Friberg et al. reported less than 2% failure rate over a 3-year period in 4600 implants.

Although it is possible to clearly identify and differentiate between a successful and a failed implant, the challenge we face centres around identifying ailing and failing implants.

## 10.4 Treatment Planning

In the preliminary stage, it is crucial to take a thorough medical, dental and social history to identify patient suitability and assess the risk of dental implant therapy.

A key objective when completing a treatment plan is to create a functional, aesthetically pleasing and maintainable prosthesis.

## 10.5 The Key Points

1. Thorough examination of remaining hard tissues, teeth and bone.
2. Assessment of soft tissues and tissue biotype.
3. Radiographic assessment—2D/3D.
4. Study models and treatment mock-up.
5. Guide manufacture, radiographic and surgical.

6. Biomechanical requirements to analyse the stress forces. Jaw relationship, crown implant proportion and parafunction.
7. Type of prosthesis and loading—immediate, provisional or definitive.
8. Patient selection.

It is recommended that immediate loading should be avoided or carried out with extreme caution, following a comprehensive consent process, in the patients that fall into the following categories: medically compromised, smokers, severe parafunctional habits and a lack of keratinised mucosa.

## 10.6 Management of Complications and Failures

### 10.6.1 Surgical Complications

1. Instrument breakage of drill.
2. Excessive insertion torque, usually 70 NM correct and above. There is also a risk of insertion device fracture.
3. Insufficient insertion torque, spinning implants.
4. Haemorrhage—especially in patients on anticoagulants such as aspirin. Soft-tissue bleeds are easily controlled with local measures such as pressure. Management of arterial and venous haemorrhage requires methods such as clamping and electrocoagulation. Damage to the sublingual artery by perforation of the mandibular lingual plates is a serious and life-threatening condition, and the patient *must* be referred to a specialised

A & E department immediately. Injury to the palatine or nasopalatine vessels must be plugged or tied off if possible.

### 10.6.2 Nerve Injuries

Judicious pre-operative planning will avoid damage to the inferior alveolar nerve. 3D scanning should be considered as the gold standard. To avoid damage to the mental nerve, careful dissection to identify its origin is essential when working in this area. Should the operator find that they have transgressed the neurovascular bundle of the inferior dental canal at the time of implant placement, then the implant should be immediately removed.

### 10.6.3 Bone Fenestration and Dehiscence

This can be managed with a variety of guided bone-regenerative procedures.

### 10.6.4 Damage to the Neighbouring Teeth

Correct planning and angulation of osteotomies will avoid damaging the roots of The adjacent teeth. Should such a damage occur, endodontic therapy, whether orthograde or

Retrograde, can be considered. Occasionally, tooth extraction is required. 3D planning and use of surgical guides will significantly minimise the risk.

## 10.7 Early Post-Operative Complications

### 10.7.1 Haemorrhaging and Bruising

Mild pressure to the area or mouth rinse with an adjunct such as tranexamic acid should suffice; in severe cases, a second procedure may be required.

Most bruising, if not voluminous, will disappear without intervention after around 7 days.

### 10.7.2 Oedema

The complexity and duration of a procedure is likely to influence the amount of post-operative swelling. In severe cases, it can cause the opening of the suture line.

The post-operative use of corticosteroids can significantly, in selected cases, impact any potential oedema.

### 10.7.3 Infection

In the presence of pus exudate and pain, the area should be opened, cleaned and appropriate antibiotic therapy should be prescribed. This may impact significantly on the osseointegration process.

### 10.7.4 Wound Dehiscence

Suturing the flap under tension will inevitably cause the wound to open. If the dehiscence is large, the wound must be closed again. Using chlorhexidine or an antiseptic mouthwash will encourage healing by secondary intention.

### 10.7.5 Implant Mobility

In the event that the implant becomes mobile, it should be removed.

## 10.8 Late Surgical Implications

### 10.8.1 Exposure of the Cover Screw

This is usually of no significance unless there is a high aesthetic demand. In situations with high aesthetic demands, the operator should consider soft-tissue grafting to achieve coverage and closure. This will usually occur if the implant has been placed crestally to the alveolar ridge.

### 10.8.2 Swelling Around the Healing Abutment

In these cases, usually the implant is well-integrated, but the healing abutment becomes loose. Remove the healing abutment, disinfect or place a new heling abutment, debride the tissue, and re-tighten.

### 10.8.3 Chronic Sinusitis

Where implants placed in simultaneously with a sinus lift procedure are performed incorrectly, contamination of the sinuses can leads to infection. If it persists, the implant and graft should be removed, and the patient should be referred to a specialist ENT team for a second opinion.

### 10.8.4 Swallowing or Inhaling Small Instruments or Components

The patient should be referred immediately for an x-ray or specialist treatment to remove the instrument/component.

## 10.9 Prosthetic Complications

The provision of implant dentistry is currently being provided in an atmosphere of enthusiasm and optimism on the part of the dental profession. Whilst it is impossible to guarantee success, what we can guarantee is our commitment to providing care, giving our utmost effort and being readily available to assist in the rare instance when problems do arise, and, if necessary, recognising when to refer the patient to a more qualified or experienced operator.

A publication by C.J. Goodacre related prosthetic complications to the following types of prosthesis.

1. Implant-fixed complete denture
2. Implant-retained overdenture
3. Implant-fixed partial prosthesis
4. Implant-supported single crowns

Complications reported as a percentage of frequency of occurrence

| Implant-Fixed Complete Denture/Bridge Complications | | |
|---|---|---|
| 1. | Denture tooth/veneer fracture | 28% |
| 2. | Screw-access hole filling material lost | 25% |
| 3. | Denture tooth wear | 15% |
| 4. | Fracture of ceramic/porcelain veneer | 12% |
| 5. | Soft-tissue hyperplasia | 9% |
| 6. | Framework fracture | 5% |
| 7. | Abutment screw fracture | 2% |
| 8. | Prosthesis screw loosening | 1% |

| 3.7b | Implant-Retained Overdenture Complications | |
|---|---|---|
| 1. | Overdenture adjustment | 92% |
| 2. | Attachment replacement | 90% |
| 3. | Reactivation of attachment | 53% |
| 4. | Mucosal Hyperplasia | 31% |
| 5. | Overdenture reline | 26% |
| 6. | Opposing denture reline | 25% |
| 7. | Loose attachment | 18% |
| 8. | Occlusal adjustment | 18% |
| 9. | Overdenture repair | 14% |
| 10. | Overdenture remake | 12% |
| 11. | Denture tooth fracture | 12% |
| 12. | Extension bar fractures | 0% |
| 13. | Overdenture fracture | 9% |
| 14. | Bar screw loosening | 6% |
| 15. | Bar fractures | 6% |
| 16. | Attachment fractures/loss | 5% |
| 17. | Excessive denture tooth wear | 4% |

| 3.7c | Fixed-Implant Partial Prosthesis Complications | |
|---|---|---|
| 1. | Porcelain veneer fracture | 6% |
| 2. | Loss of retention—cement-retained | 6% |
| 3. | Screw loosening of screw-retained prosthesis | 4% |
| 4. | Screw loosening with cement-retained prosthesis | 3% |

| 3.7d | Implant-Retained Single-Crown Complications | |
|---|---|---|
| 1. | Abutment screw loosening | 3% |
| 2. | Implant fracture | 3% |
| 3. | Porcelain fracture/chipping | 3% |
| 4. | Loss of retention—cement retained | 2% |
| 5. | Open proximal contacts/food impaction | 2% |
| 6. | Crown remakes | 1% |

Of the cement-retained single crowns, Korsch et al. found 59.5% have excess cement, with the resulting sequalae of peri-implantitis.

The choice of material used in the final restoration can also have a significant impact on the success of your restoration. Certain materials and techniques driven by the industry can lead to catastrophic outcomes, leaving the dentist and dental technician responsible for resolving the resulting issues. Zirconium oxide is an example of a material that is currently being lauded as the replacement for metal. The material is a great choice of material in many clinical indications, but its processing and sintering is very technique-sensitive. The material shrinks by up to 20% during sintering; its use in a full-arch restoration presents some real challenges in achieving passivity of fit.

## 10.10 Conclusions

1. Implant overdentures present with more complications overall, with the maintenance taking up considerable chair time.
2. Single-implant, cement- or screw-retained crowns present the lowest number of complications.
3. The most common complication/complaint with implant-fixed complete prosthesis was tooth fracture.
4. The most common complication associated with implant-retained overdentures is the need for adjustments and component fracture.
5. Porcelain veneer fractures are the most common complication found in implant retained fixed prosthesis.
6. The most common problems occurring with implant-retained single crowns is the abutment screw loosening and the management of excess cement.

Implant-supported overdentures present with more complications than implant-supported fixed prosthesis, full or partial and single-tooth implant-supported crowns.

The lowest complication rate is reported with single-tooth implants, with the most common complication being loosening of the screw or cement element.

The overall success or failure criteria for a dental implant are extremely difficult to describe, as is the care for natural teeth. The range from health to disease is similar for both. The primary criteria for assessing quality are pain and mobility. The successful management of dental implants relies on meticulous diagnostic treatment planning and the surgical/prosthetic skills of the operator.

With any biomechanical entity, difficulties can arise in the area of biological function as well as mechanical or engineered stability.

## Further Reading

Aperilli M, Abundo R, Corrente G, Saccone C. Short (5 and 7 mm long) porous implants in the posterior atrophic maxilla: a 5-year report of a prospective single cohort study. Eur J Oral Implantol. 2012;5:265–72.

Cakarer S, Can T, Yaltirik M, Keskin C. Complications associated with the ball, bar and locator attachments for implant supported overdentures. Med Oral Patol Oral Cir Bucal. 2011;16:e953–9.

Esposito M, Maghaireh H, Pistilli R, Grusovin G, Lee ST, Trullenque-Erikson A, Gualini F. Dental implants with internal vs external connections: 5-year post-loading results from a pragmatic multicenter randomized controlled trial. Eur J Oral Implantol. 2016;9:129–41.

Fathima M, Sinha N, Ali SM. Failures in dental implants: a review. Int J Adv Health Sci. 2017;4(2):5–9.

Francetti L, Corbella S, Taschieri S, Cavalli N, Fabbro M. Medium- and long-term complications in full arch rehabilitations supported by upright and tilted implants. Clin Implant Dent Relat Res. 2015;17:758–64.

Gibbard LL, Zarb G. A 5-year prospective study of implant supported single tooth replacements. J Can Dent Assoc. 2002;68:110–6.

Gothberg C, Bergendal T, Magnusson T. Complications after treatment with implant supported fixed prostheses, a retrospective study. Int J Prosthodont. 2003;16:201–7.

Gotfredsen K. A 10-year prospective study of single tooth implants placed in the anterior maxilla. Clin Implant Dent Relat Res. 2012;14:80–7.

Goodacre BJ, Goodacre SE, Goodacre CJ. Prosthetic complications with implant prosthesis (2001–2017). Eur J Oral Implantol. 2018;11(Suppl 1):S27–36.

Goodacre CJ, Bernal G, Rungcharassaeng K, Kan JY. Summary common complication with implants and implant prostheses. J Prosthet Dent. 2003;90:121–32. Review/Dental Implants.

Grandi T, Guazzi P, Samarani R, Garuti G, Grandi G. Immediate loading of two unsplinted implants retaining the existing complete mandibular denture in elderly edentulous patients: 1-year results from a multicenter prospective cohort study. Eur J Oral Implantol. 2012;5:61–8.

Gunne J, Jemt T, Linden B. Implant treatment in partially edentulous patients: a report on prostheses after 3 years. Int J Prosthodont. 1994;7:143–8.

Jemt T, Johansson J. Implant treatment in the edentulous maxillae: 1 15 year follow up study on 76 consecutive patients provided with fixed prostheses. Clin Implant Dent Relat Res. 2006;8:61–9.

Jemt T. Cemented CeraOne and porcelain fused to TiAdapt abutment single implant crown restorations: a 10-year comparative follow up study. Clin Implant Dent Relat Res. 2009;11:303–10.

Karthik K, Sivakumar S, Thangaswarmy V. Evaluation of implant success: a review of past and present concepts. J Pharm BioAllied Sci. 2013;5(Suppl 1):S117–9.

Malo P, de Araujo NM, Lopes A, Queridinha B, Ferro A, Gravito I. Axial implants in immediate function for partial rehabilitation in the maxilla and mandible: a retrospective clinical study evaluating the long term outcome (up to 10 years). Implant Dent. 2015;24:557–64.

Mangano C, Mangano F, Shibli JA, Ricci M, Sammons RL, Figliuzzi M. Morse taper connection implants supporting 'planned' maxillary and mandibular bar retained overdentures: a 5-year prospective multicenter study. Clin Oral Implants Res. 2011;22:1117–24.

Meijer HJA, Geertman ME, Raghoebar GM, Kwakman JM. Implant retained mandibular overdentures: 6-year results of a multicenter clinical trial on 3 different implant systems. J Oral Maxillofac Surg. 2001;59:1260–8.

Prashanti E, Sajjan S, Reddy JM. Failures in implants. Indian J Dent Res. 2011;22(3):446–53.

Popat RP, Bhavsar NV, Popat PR. Peri-implantitis: management of ailing, failing and failed dental implants. IOSR J Dent Med Sci. 2014;13(1, Ver. VIII):43–6. p-ISSN: 2279-0853, p-ISSN: 2279-0861.

Quirynen M, Naert I, van Steenberghe D, Dekeyser C, Callens A. Periodontal aspects of osseointegrated fixtures supporting a partial bridge. An up to 6 years retrospective study. J Clin Periodontol. 1992;19:118–26.

Schwarz S, Schroder C, Corcodel N, Hassel AJ, Rammelsberg P. Retrospective comparison of semi-permanent and permanent cementation of implant supported single crowns and FDP's with regard to the incidence of survival and complications. Clin Implant Dent Relat Res. 2012;14:e151–8.

Simon R. Single implant supported molar and pre-molar crowns: a ten-year retrospective clinical report. J Prosthet Dent. 2003;90:517–21.

Verma AK, Mariyam A, Pratibha K, Abhishek G, Naeem A, Kumar TA. Success and failure of dental implants. Int J Adv Dent Res. 2016;1(1):01–4.

Wennstrom JL, Ekestubbe A, Grondahl K, Karlsson S, Lindhe J. Implant supported single tooth restorations: a 5-year prospective study. J Clin Periodontol. 2005;32:567–74.

Widbom C, Soderfeldt B, Kronstrom M. A retrospective evaluation of treatments with implant supported maxillary overdentures. Clin Implant Dent Relat Res. 2005;7:166–72.

Zweers J, Doornik Av Hogendorf EAH, Quirynen M, Van der Weijden GA. Clinical and radiography evaluation of narrow vs regular diameter dental implants: a 3 year follow up. A retrospective study. Clin Oral Implants Res. 2015;26:149–56.

# Implant Diseases

# 11

Craig Barclay

Why implants fail and when they fail may be a good way to consider the topic of dental implant disease.

Failure of a dental implant can be:

- Early: No integration.
- Late: Integration has occurred and something subsequently causes bone loss

Early failure is often related to implant surgery or post-surgery infection or the occurrence of micro-motion during the healing phase of implant placement.

Therefore, following this train of thought, implant diseases are associated with late implant failure.

It is vital to understand that peri-implant diseases develop and destroy soft tissue and bone much more rapidly than is the case with periodontitis. Moreover, it should be considered that peri-implantitis is more difficult to treat than periodontitis.

**Peri-implant mucositis** is an inflammatory lesion affecting the marginal soft tissues that surround osseo-integrated dental implants, and is induced by the accumulation of a plaque biofilm or other conditions; this does not involve inflammatory resorption of the bone (Fig. 11.1).

**Peri-implantitis** is an inflammatory lesion affecting the tissues (hard and/or soft) surrounding osseo-integrated dental implants, induced or propagated by the accumulation of a plaque biofilm or other conditions, and which involves progressive inflammatory resorption of the supporting bone. It is recognised that bone loss around an osseo-integrated dental implant may result from causes other than inflammation (Figs. 11.2 and 11.3).

---

C. Barclay (✉)
Restorative Dentistry/Oral Rehabilitation, Manchester Foundation Trust, Manchester, UK
e-mail: craig.barclay@mft.nhs.uk



C. Barclay (ed.), *Oral Implantology: Assessment to Maintenance*, BDJ Clinician's Guides, https://doi.org/10.1007/978-3-031-55241-0_11

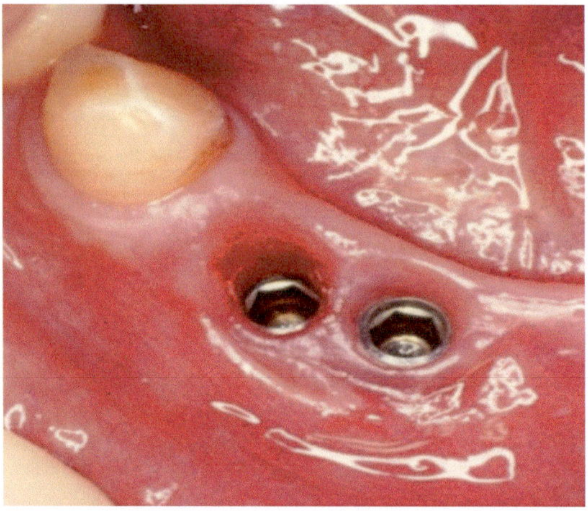

**Fig. 11.1** Peri-implant mucositis with marked inflammation and bleeding from around the abutment collar of the dental implant

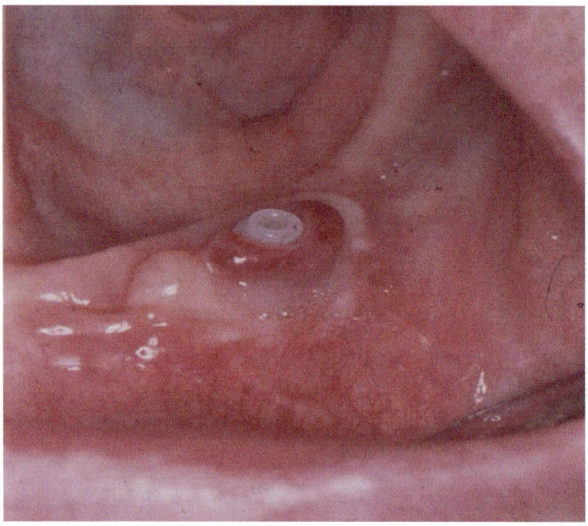

**Fig. 11.2** Clinical presentation of an inflamed collar around a dental implant that often has associated bone loss

**Retrograde peri-implantitis** is defined as a clinically symptomatic peri-apical lesion (diagnosed as a radiolucency) that develops shortly after implant insertion while the coronal portion of the implant achieves a normal bone-to-implant interface (Fig. 11.4).

Peri-implant diseases are generally considered to be inflammatory conditions affecting the soft and hard gum tissues around dental implants. Dental implants are titanium-coated surfaces in a fluid oral environment and, therefore, a biofilm forms rapidly. The bacterial colonisation of this biofilm and its management will, to some extent, influence the long-term survival of that dental implant fixture.

Therefore, some of the factors that have been suggested as potential risk indicators for peri-implant mucositis include biofilm accumulation, smoking and radiation, diabetes, lack of keratinised mucosa, obesity and presence of excess luting cement [1].

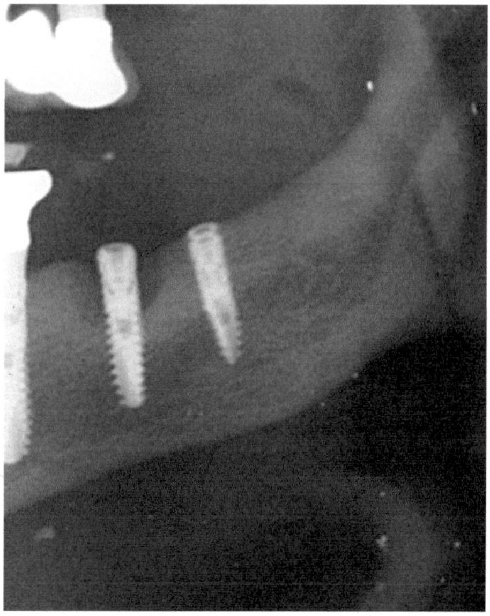

**Fig. 11.3** Crater bony defect around a dental implant

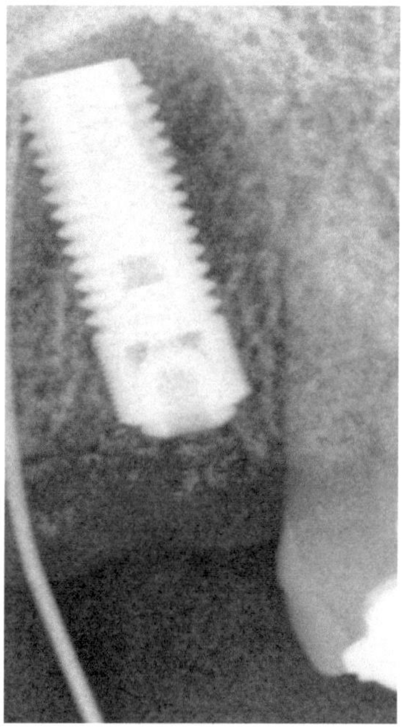

**Fig. 11.4** Retrograde peri-implantitis with an associated sinus tract and apical radiolucency, which resolved after a course of antibiotics

What is the risk for conversion from peri-implant mucositis to peri-implantitis?

There is some evidence on the patient level from a retrospective study that the lack of annual supportive therapy in patients diagnosed with peri-implant mucositis was associated with increased risk for conversion of mucositis to peri-implantitis

[2]. In a five-year follow-up, 18% of the patients who had supportive maintenance implant therapy presented with peri-implantitis, while 43.9% of patients who had no supportive therapy developed peri-implantitis. The histopathological and clinical conditions resulting in the conversion of peri-implant mucositis to peri-implantitis are not completely understood.

The term 'peri-implantitis' first appeared in a study by Mombelli et al. [3]. Peri-implantitis has been defined as a 'plaque-associated pathologic condition occurring in the tissue around dental implants, characterized by inflammation in the peri-implant mucosa and subsequent progressive loss of supporting bone'. Subsequent to the proceedings of the first European Workshop on Periodontology (EWP), Albrektsson and Isidor presented definitions for two peri-implant disease entities, peri-implant mucositis and peri-implantitis, in a consensus report [4]. Modified definitions were published after the sixth EWP to include the collective term peri-implant disease. However, the problem exists when both the following situations are defined as peri-implantitis: the classical crater defect seen in Fig. 11.3, and an anterior dental implant placed in a narrow width of bone which progressively loses the buccal plate, but retains the mesial and distal bone height. Clearly, these are two distinct disease entities with different underlying causative factors, but both are described in the literature as peri-implantitis (Albrektsson et al. [5], Fig. 11.5).

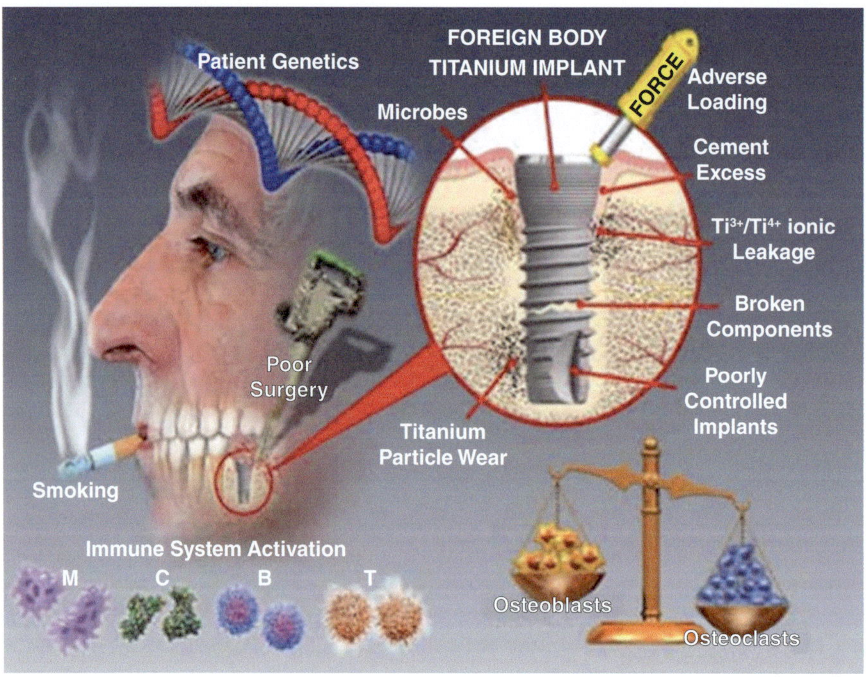


**Fig. 11.5** A series of factors work together to activate the immune system, ultimately leading to a shift in the balance between osteoblastic and osteoclastic activity, resulting in bone loss

The incidence of peri-implant mucositis and peri-implantitis in the population is widely debated.

In one study, the incidence of peri-implant mucositis at the patient level was 51.9% after 5 years of evaluation and 57.0% after 10 years. Incidence of peri-implantitis at the patient level was 16.9% after 5 years of evaluation and 29.7% after 10 years [6].

Another study suggested peri-implant mucositis occurs in about 80% of subjects (50% of sites) restored with implants, and peri-implantitis in between 28% and 56% of subjects (12%–40% of sites). Lindhe and Meyle, on behalf of Group D of the European Workshop on Periodontology [7]

A further study suggested the prevalence of peri-implantitis to be 6.61% over a 9- to 14-year period [8].

The challenge is of course to know which of these studies to believe in terms of how you manage your patients who receive dental implants and what advice you give them in terms of the longevity of this treatment modality and the likely incidence of peri-implant disease that may affect them during their clinical history. As with all disease processes, the balance between health and disease is influenced by many factors, and, therefore, patients who are deemed to have a higher risk of developing dental implant diseases should be recalled and maintained with a shorter recall interval than those patients who have fewer risk factors.

An important factor for the long-term success of dental implants is the maintenance of healthy peri-implant tissues. Therefore methodical and thorough assessment of a dental implant when monitoring peri-implant tissues is essential. There should be a recording of an initial clinical baseline assessment and a radiographic record of baseline bone levels. Dental implants show a small amount of bone loss within the first year of function, and then lesser amounts of physiological bone loss with time. Therefore, the foundation of a successful implant therapy is optimal oral hygiene practiced by the patient at home, and professional maintenance support plays a vital role in this process. This involves the professional removal of biofilm and associated oral pathogens. Some of these pathogens are associated with periodontal disease; however, dentate patients face a different biofilm challenge compared to those with implants are placed in the edentulous mouth.

The use of various mechanical methods to remove biofilm from the implant surface has been debated in the literature. The use of titanium scalers and curettes and linear action piezoelectric titanium tips for biofilm removal has been advocated [9]. Certainly, these methods are less likely to produce heat compared to cavitron tips. Air flow/perio flow with erythitol powder [10] delivers a systematic and predictable professional prophylaxis around dental implants and their bridgework restorations and can rapidly remove biofilm painlessly both supra- and subgingivally.

In terms of home care, air/water flossing machines can be utilised to modify biofilm is may help prevent peri-mucositis and peri-implantitis.

The use of mouthwashes to disrupt this biofilm may be a useful adjunct such as chlorhexidine digluconate, which has a broad-spectrum antimicrobial spectrum against gram positive and gram-negative pathogens. Essential oils mouthwashes the scientific liteature suggest have a greater reduction in plaque biofilm [11, 12] than with mechanical methods or chlorhexidine—affecting the maturation of the biofilm on the implant surface.

The importance of keratinised mucosa in the long-term maintenance of peri-implant health is debated [13]. The evidence is equivocal; however, keratinised mucosa may have advantages regarding patient comfort and ease of plaque removal.

It is, therefore, suggested that implant therapy must not be limited purely to the placement and restoration of dental implants but should be extended to the implementation of peri-implant maintenance therapy to prevent biologic complications and hence to increase the likelihood of long-term success. This therapy must be tailored to a patient's risk profiling, but findings suggest that a minimum recall interval of 5 to 6 months is advocated. Peri-implant maintenance therapy does not eliminate the risk of biological complications; therefore, all patient-related, clinical, and implant-related risk factors must be explored thoroughly.

## References

1. Heitz-Mayfield LJA, Salvi GE. Peri-implant mucositis. J Clin Periodontol. 2018;45(Suppl 20):S237–45.
2. Costa FO, Takenaka-Martinez S, Cota LOM, Ferreira SD, Silva GLM, Costa JE. Peri-implant disease in subjects with and without preventive maintenance: a 5-year follow-up. J Clin Periodontol. 2012;39(2):173–81.
3. Mombelli A, van Oosten MA, Schurch E Jr, Land NP. The microbiota associated with successful or failing osseointegrated titanium implants. Oral Microbiol Immunol. 1987;2(4):145–51.
4. Albrektsson T, Isidor F. Consensus report of session IV. In: Lang NP, Karring T, editors. Proceedings of the first European workshop on periodontology. London: Quintessence Publishing; 1994. p. 365–9.
5. Albrektsson T, Canullo L, Cochran D, De Bruyn H. "Peri-implantitis": a complication of a foreign body or a man-made "disease". Facts and fiction. Clin Implant Dent Relat Res. 2016;18(4):840–9.
6. Meijer HJA, Raghoebar GM, de Waal YCM, Vissink A. Incidence of peri-implant mucositis and peri-implantitis in edentulous patients with an implant-retained mandibular overdenture during a 10-year follow-up period. J Clin Periodontol. 2014;41(12):1178–83.
7. Lindhe J, Meyle J. Peri-implant diseases: consensus report of the sixth European workshop on periodontology. J Clin Periodontol. 2008;35(8 Suppl):282–5.
8. Roos-Jansåker AM, Lindahl C, Renvert H, Renvert S. Nine- to fourteen-year follow-up of implant treatment. Part II: presence of peri-implant lesions. J Clin Periodontol. 2006;33(4):290–5.
9. Nee WY, Awang RAR, Hassan A. Effects on the titanium implant surface by different hygiene instrumentations: a narrative review. Cureus. 2022;14(10):e30884.
10. Amate-Fernández P, Figueiredo R, Blanc V, Àlvarez G, León R, Valmaseda-Castellón E. Erythritol-enriched powder and oral biofilm regrowth on dental implants: an in vitro study. Med Oral Patol Oral Cir Bucal. 2021;26(5):e602.
11. Esposito M, Worthington HV, Thomsen P, Coulthard P. Interventions for replacing missing teeth: maintaining health around dental implants. Cochrane Database Syst Rev. 2004;3:CD003069. https://doi.org/10.1002/14651858.CD003069.pub2.
12. Heasman P, Esmail Z, Barclay C. Peri-implant diseases. Dent Update. 2010;37(8):511–2, 514–6.
13. Mahardawi B, Jiaranuchart S, Damrongsirirat N, Arunjaroensuk S, Mattheos N, Somboonsavatdee A, Pimkhaokham A. The lack of keratinized mucosa as a risk factor for peri-implantitis: a systematic review and meta-analysis. Sci Rep. 2023;13(1):3778.

# Index




C. Barclay (ed.), *Oral Implantology: Assessment to Maintenance*, BDJ Clinician's Guides, https://doi.org/10.1007/978-3-031-55241-0

MIX
Papier aus verantwortungsvollen Quellen
Paper from responsible sources
FSC® C105338

If you have any concerns about our products,
you can contact us on
**ProductSafety@springernature.com**

In case Publisher is established outside the EU,
the EU authorized representative is:
**Springer Nature Customer Service Center GmbH**
**Europaplatz 3, 69115 Heidelberg, Germany**

Printed by Libri Plureos GmbH
in Hamburg, Germany